Eighty-Seven Thyroid Disease Questions Answered!

Self-Educate through Hypothyroid and Hyperthyroid Q & A!

By: James M. Lowrance © 2010

Eighty-Seven Thyroid Disease Questions Answered!

TABLE OF CONTENTS:

SECTION ONE: Questions and Answers ONE through FIFTEEN

SECTION TWO: Questions and Answers SIXTEEN through THIRTY

SECTION THREE: Questions and Answers THIRTY-ONE through FOURTY-FIVE

SECTION FOUR: Questions and Answers FOURTY-SIX through SIXTY

SECTION FIVE: Questions and Answers SIXTY-ONE through SEVENTY-FIVE

SECTION SIX: Questions and Answers SEVENTY-SIX through EIGHTY-SEVEN

Eighty-Seven Thyroid Disease Questions Answered!

INTRODUCTION:

This book is derived from forum post replies Jim Lowrance made to fellow thyroid patients on a number of community websites, over the course of approximately 5 years (between the years 2004 to 2009). These replies were in regard to many thyroid disease issues, including difficulties adjusting to thyroid hormone replacement for hypothyroidism, anxiety and depression that can occur in treated hyperthyroid and hypothyroid patients, peripheral and autonomic neuropathy symptoms of thyroid disease, co-morbid adrenal fatigue, thyroid removal surgeries and procedures and many other highly concerning aspects of living with thyroid disease.

While Jim has tweaked these answers he posted just a bit so that they flow well for the readers or listeners of them, in most cases he left them relatively the same as they were originally posted and in so doing, they convey the sense of discussion that occurred between fellow thyroid patients who can learn from shared personal experiences. While Jim only includes his own side of these discussions, he does state at the beginning of each reply made, the general questions that were asked by thyroid patients seeking answers for problems they were experiencing.

Eighty-Seven Thyroid Disease Questions Answered!

Certainly these discussions were not intended to replace the instructions and treatments of doctors but rather to help thyroid patients become better educated about their diseases, so that they become increasingly proactive in their treatments while staying partnered with their treating doctors. Jim would highly suggest this same attitude for those who read or hear the information in this compiled information resource because it is important to always recognize your medical doctor as your most important avenue toward an improved quality of life but to also recognize the benefits of becoming a well informed thyroid patent.

-Jim Lowrance

SECTION ONE:
Questions and Answers ONE through FIFTEEN

QUESTION ONE

Have you had Personal Experience with Thyrotoxicity - Overtreated Hypothyroidism?

Yes and I recently posted on a thyroid forum, in regard to being found in a state of over treated hypothyroidism. Following is my descriptive post in regard to this issue and how it is being resolved. ---

"Something has come up in the area of my hypothyroid treatment via Armour thyroid brand, combination - T4/T3 medication.

You will be blown away when you hear what my current blood levels are because I should be bouncing off the walls with hyperthyroid symptoms. Instead, I'm mainly fatigued, with stressed-out feelings. I do have muscle weakness and have been seeing a neurologist due to a few more sensory and tingling symptoms of aching, occasional stabbing pains etc... I had some low amplitude readings on an EMG.

Eighty-Seven Thyroid Disease Questions Answered!

It's possible any nerve damage I have will be helped via the fact I was also found vitamin deficient in D, E and insufficient (low normal) in B12, which are all now being treated.

Now to my blood labs - (ready for this?)---

My TSH result was at "0.05" - Range 0.25 to 5.00 [TSH drops below normal with hyperthyroidism]

My FT3 was a whopping "903" - Range 210 to 440 [it elevates with hyperthyroidism]

My Total T3 was nearly as bad (I prefer the "free levels" to be tested). It was @ "365" - Range 76 to 181 [which is also also at hyperthyroid level for T3]

Both T3s were more than TWICE the highest normal cut off value! In spite of this, my Dr.s Office called and said my levels were only "a little high" and in fact they were going to place me on a DOSE INCREASE prior to seeing these results, because I have gained a little weight since my last visit and my T4 was actually on the low-side, which has been typical of how my "Armour Thyroid" brand of hormone therapy manifests on my labs for the many years I've been treated with it.

Eighty-Seven Thyroid Disease Questions Answered!

It was I who demanded my T3 be tested because they kept failing to add it on my lab requisitions, even with my repeated requests and I had a suspicion the levels were high.

Can a person have these high of levels and not actually feel like their metabolism is sped up (hyperthyroid)?

Regardless, I know it is very unwise to maintain this type level due to risk of bone loss and possible heart rhythm complications. I'm now also beginning to wonder if my high levels of T3 have contributed to my muscle weakness and peripheral neuropathy type symptoms (I feel it is likely not the cause, since I began experiencing these symptoms long before the over-treated hypothyroidism)!

In defense of the doctor, I will say that she had not yet seen the T3 result when she recommended the dose increase but she based the idea on my T4 which was at "0.8" in the range of 0.9 to 1.8 ng/dL (flagged as being slightly low). My disappointment with the doctor is in the fact that a former MD I went to, who discontinued his practice due to a back problem, told me that T3 was important to test when taking the Armour Thyroid brand of hormone replacement.

I told the new doctor this, at my first visit with her back in February 2010 but she kept failing to add the test on my thyroid panels. I made sure it was added this time, by kicking and screaming a little and sure enough I'm over-treated.

I'm currently taking 2.5 grains, so will reduce it back to 2 grains and hopefully this will be enough of a decrease between now and when I get back in to a doctor (NOTE: Since writing this particular forum post, I conferred with my doctor who agreed with the dose decrease and is monitoring it with follow-up blood retests)."

QUESTION TWO

Can Neuropathy and Myopathy Occur in Thyroid Disease?

The U.S.-NIH/National Library of Medicine allows quoting of medical research published on their site (PubMed), for educational purposes and all of the quotes that will follow, are from their site, with exception of the short quote I've added by the AAFP (American Academy of Family Physicians).

Eighty-Seven Thyroid Disease Questions Answered!

I thought this might be of interest for hypothyroid patients like me. It shows that endocrine disorders in addition to diabetes are strongly associated with neurological disorders and symptoms.

(Note: In some studies, neuropathies did not resolve or only did-so partially in 'treated' hypothyroid patients and in my opinion, this is likely the case more often in <u>autoimmune cases</u> of hypothyroidism.)

(American Academy of Family Physicians): "Muscle weakness is a common complaint among patients presenting to the family physician's office. Although the cause of weakness occasionally may be apparent, often it is unclear, puzzling the physician and frustrating the patient."

1. **Pain and small-fiber neuropathy in patients with hypothyroidism** (U.S. National Library of Medicine – PubMed) --- "Conclusions: Some patients treated for hypothyroidism have symptoms and findings compatible with small-fiber neuropathy or "hyper phenomena" indicating central sensitization. ...of Eighteen patients...Eight were classified as having large fiber neuropathy..."

Eighty-Seven Thyroid Disease Questions Answered!

2. **Hypothyroidism and polyneuropathy.** (U.S. National Library of Medicine – PubMed) --- "Using standard electrophysiological criteria, a definite diagnosis of polyneuropathy was made in 28 cases (72%). The commonest sites of abnormal nerve conduction were the sensory nerves, especially the sural nerve."

3. **Hypothyroid neuropathy and myopathy: clinical and electrodiagnostic longitudinal findings.** (U.S. National Library of Medicine – PubMed) --- "This case shows that thyroid hormone replacement eliminates the neuropathic manifestations of severe hypothyroidism. In contrast, the myopathic features, such as weakness and muscle wasting, may persist despite maintenance of the euthyroid state."

4. **Neuromuscular status of thyroid diseases: a prospective clinical and electrodiagnostic study.** (U.S. National Library of Medicine – PubMed) --- Among the thyroid patients, 17 (42.5%) patients were diagnosed with mononeuropathy and polyneuropathy. Entrapment neuropathy was observed in 30% and diffuse neuropathy in 10% of the patients. Myopathy findings were observed in 2 patients.

5. **Aspects of peripheral nerve involvement in patients with treated hypothyroidism.** (U.S. National Library of Medicine – PubMed) --- "RESULTS: Sixty-three per cent of the patients with 'pure' hypothyroidism had abnormalities on NCS, 25% had reduced IENF density and 31% had abnormalities on QST. Four patients (25%) met criteria for small fibre polyneuropathy, the other (75%) were classified as having mixed fiber polyneuropathy.

QUESTION THREE

Any Symptom Trouble Shooting Suggestions for Thyroid Patients?

I was diagnosed with Hashimoto's thyroiditis and hypothyroidism in 2003, at about age-40. I do also have dysautonomia -- imbalance in my involuntary nervous system but I've never asked for a tilt-test. It is a test that detects abnormal blood pressure imbalances with postural changes, revealing dysautonomia. I know for a fact it's there however and has been since my teen years.

Eighty-Seven Thyroid Disease Questions Answered!

I want to mention some things I had tested, that might give leads to fellow thyroid patients, whose treatments failed to resolve certain types of symptoms they were experiencing.

Due to my unresolved fatigue, muscle weakness and neuro-type symptoms (despite treatment for hypothyroidism), one board certified MD suggested that I have comorbid (co-occurring) Chronic Fatigue Syndrome (CFS) because I have apparent immuno-deficiency including allergies (i.e. thyroid autoimmunity and persistent asthma). In the case of CFS however, one must rule out all other possible causes of unresolved symptoms, to arrive at a diagnosis.

I believe, among many other things, one should have vitamin levels tested, such as B12, B6, D and E because each of these can negatively affect the nervous system if deficient but the problem is usually easily reversed with supplementation of deficient vitamins. I was found deficient in D and E and insufficient (low normal) in B12. I had my doctor test me for kidney/liver levels and anti-mitochondrial antibodies (AMA), to make sure my malabsorption was not due to kidney or liver problems.

I do have fatty liver (I'm moderately overweight) but no biliary involvement or hepatitis (serious liver diseases). It doesn't hurt to rule these out if one is diagnosed with deficiencies of fat-soluble vitamins (the ones previously mentioned).

Another fact to discuss with a qualified doctor, is the fact that "thyroid antibodies" can be present/positive before thyroid hormone levels become imbalanced, so if these haven't been tested-for, this might be something to also consider if one is experiencing unexplainable symptoms. According to the U.S. NIH (PubMed), thyroid antibodies can cause symptoms even when the person affected is in a euthroid state (normal hormone levels).

I also feel that symptoms can also point to the need for a person's sex hormones to be tested and these can be affected if adrenal hormones are low, such as pregnenolone and DHEA which convert into sex hormones as the body needs them (male-androgens and female-progesterones, which both sexes have in different balances). I personally have also had adrenal fatigue since 2003 or earlier and repeat saliva and urinary cortisol tests showed mine to be low but DHEA was always normal or even high-normal.

Eighty-Seven Thyroid Disease Questions Answered!

Adrenal saliva test kits can now be obtained through local pharmacies or online and medical research has proven these to be accurate. I've always felt that lack of immunity (immune system dysfunction), dysautonomia (nervous system imbalances) and endocrine dysfunction (problems in hormone-producing glands) are all tied closely together. One imbalance of a system can affect one or all of the others. These are just a few suggestions for trouble-shooting unresolved symptoms in treated thyroid patients.

QUESTION FOUR

We Know Hypothyroid Treatment is not perfect but is it Essential?

I'm one of the rare male hypothyroid patients with Hashimoto's thyroiditis. Just this year, I was finally tested for vitamin deficiencies and my D was also deficient at: "17" (range 30 to 100). My B12 was lower-normal (insufficient), so I'm treated for both it and the D with replacement mega-dose vitamins.

Eighty-Seven Thyroid Disease Questions Answered!

15

I went to a neurologist-specialist due to long-term muscle weakness and easy fatigability, that I was convinced since 2004, was CFS (chronic Fatigue Syndrome), comorbid to my thyroid disease. He had the forethought to also check my vitamin E, since my D was deficient and B12 was insufficient and "Presto!" it was deficient as well, at: "0.4" (range 3.0 to 15.8) - in fact, being at less than half a point, it was likely my worst deficiency.

I've been active as a patient advocate since diagnosis and my occasional difficulty with some doctors - such as my current over-treatment on thyroid hormone replacement for hypothyroidism (my blood work showed my T3 to be more than double highest normal range). -- are the type things that, that we patients should look out for (pro-activeness).

Anyway, I mainly try to dispel the imbalanced opinion (kindly, diplomatically and politely), that suggests thyroid hormone replacement is perfect in all cases and fixes all the problems thyroid patients have within weeks of being administered. Don't get me wrong -- I thank God for thyroid hormone therapy and for doctors who are compassionate and attentive.

However, without patient proactive-ness in their treatments, things can most certainly go wrong, regardless of a doctor's expertise or a thyroid hormone brand's effectiveness. There can also be comorbid (co-occurring) disorders like vitamin deficiencies or a number of other things that also need to be diagnosed and treated.

So... My message since 2003 to fellow patients is to become self-educated, best possible, via good, reliable sources and to be proactive in treatment and to partner with their doctors if at all possible!

QUESTION FIVE

Any Association between Dysautonomia and Thyroid Disease?

I believe there is an association between these two health disorders and I'll give my personal experience as an example: I have had orthostatic hypotension since my teens - a common form of dysautonomia.

Mine is the type that only causes me the weird pressure sensation in my head and neck due to a short episode of blood pressure drop, when I first stand-up but I've never had syncope with it (fainting). Rarely when I was younger I would experience a drop-out of my vision for just a couple seconds. In-short, with my other symptoms of chronic fatigue, generalized anxiety etc..., I believe I'm likely in the POTS (Postural Orthostatic Tachycardia Syndrome) or in the MVPS (Mitral Valve Prolapse Syndrome - common heart murmur) category.

I also have Hashimoto's/hypothyroidism, which I understand to be a common finding in dysautonomic patients and in those with MVP and in the past few months I was found deficient in 2 vitamins (E and D) and insufficient/low-normal in a third one (B12) - all being treated. I also believe due to my symptoms for many years of heart skips, flutters (less frequent than they used to be) and extreme sensitivity to caffeine, chocolate and alcohol, that I also have Mitral Valve Prolapse, even though my EKG was normal in 2001 (I was having frequent symptoms back then). I've not had an echocardiogram, which is sound wave imaging of my heart but I don't really feel I need one to confirm MVP because it runs in my family.

I just had EMG/Nerve Conduction studies done this year (2010) due to worsening of carpal tunnel (hand/wrist) and tarsal tunnel type problems (feet) and general muscle weakness. Part of this is likely a result of my vitamin deficiencies but because of my tendency toward anxiety/worry I became neurotically concerned about having ALS, MS or some other terrible disease. I will say in regard to my fear about muscle weakness, that I've had it far too long to be caused by a neuromuscular motor neuron disease, unless it is the slowest developing, least-aggressive type (none like this exist as far as I know). I can remember posting on forums about my muscle weakness in 2004/2005 and these posts still exist out there somewhere. I actually remember as far back as 2002 having these same type muscle symptoms and my thyroid treatment that began in 2003 never resolved them, leading me to think I had comorbid CFS (Chronic Fatigue Syndrome) with my hypothyroidism. I have never seen any atrophy (wasting/shrinkage) in my muscles.

QUESTION SIX

Can one be Over-Treated on Armour Thyroid Prescribed Hormone?

I was recently found to be over-treated on thyroid hormone replacement therapy as I stated in an earlier answer to a similar question, which is sometimes referred to as "dose induced throtoxicity" (hyperthyroidism). The following was my giving detail to this problem in a forum post. ---

Strangely enough, I didn't have classic thyrotoxic symptoms like tachycardia/rapid heart rate or weight loss (in fact I have difficulty losing – I'm moderately overweight) however, I can't imagine it not having affected me in some way because my last blood retest for T3 was as follows:

FT3 result - "903" (range 210 to 440) ----[This was twice highest normal + 23!]

Total T3 result - "365" (range 76 to 181) --- [twice highest normal + 3]

Before this, I was kept at highest normal on T3 and occasionally, just slightly above normal.

Eighty-Seven Thyroid Disease Questions Answered!

My TSH was always kept at near undetectable, such as "0.005".

The reason I agreed to this dose-level for about 6 years is because my T4 will actually drop slightly below normal if my TSH even rises to between 0.5 and 1.0. I felt this indicated that I instead needed some T4 added rather than increasing the Armour but none of my doctors would agree to do so, claiming it makes for too much opportunity for instability of the treatment. I had even thought years ago about switching to T4 but I feel that patients used to getting T4/T3 combo, need to continue it or risk falling into symptoms by switching to T4 only (i.e. depression) or their bodies may be slow in converting t4 into T3, due to it having been supplied for so long. Certainly this might not be the case but was something I didn't want to risk.

This is not a knock at doctors in-general, I assure you but in the area I reside-in, finding good doctors is an incredible challenge. I've heard many other people in my area express this same opinion - so I'm far from alone in it.

I got to post regarding this to a board certified endocrinologist at another thyroid forum.

I will be eager to see if he believes my myopathy (muscle weakness) might be related to the over-dosing. I'm also treated for D and E vitamin deficiencies and feel these play a factor as well but I certainly don't want an additional cause or contributor to that symptom!

Once seeing my Armour over-dose levels via blood retests, my Dr. had me cut back from 2.5 to 2.0 grains of the prescribed hormone and said she will blood retest me in 3 to 4 months but even this seems like a strange timing, since I feel 8-weeks would be better, so that it can be adjusted even further if-needed.

[NOTE: The MD at "the other thyroid forum" I mention above, did confirm to me, that over-treatment with thyroid hormone, can indeed cause or contribute to myopathy (muscle weakness)]

QUESTION SEVEN

What is the Importance of Thyroid Test Normal Values Ranges?

The following was my response to a fellow thyroid patient who was found to have a very low TSH level via blood tests. They also had a T4 test done (a major thyroid hormone) and a "T3 Uptake", which is not a measure of the T3 hormone level and is usually only useful in diagnosing thyroid disease. I mention in my reply to them, that posting results of blood tests is more useful for getting comments on, if the normal values reference ranges are also included. ---

"Your TSH is near undetectable and decreases to low levels with hyperthyroidism (overactive thyroid). Your T4 test might be flagged high as well but if you could post the normal range for comparison, that would help. The T3 Uptake is not always helpful (actually a measure of available globulins, that make T3 work in the body) but if you could also post the range for it and the FTI Index, this would also help since labs differ in normal values ranges.

If your doctor is having a thyroid ultrasound done on you, this is to see if you have abnormal textures in your gland. It can also detect nodules (small tumors) that can cause your thyroid to overproduce hormone if they are "hot" - meaning they are acting as if they have become thyroid tissue - absorbing iodine and manufacturing, putting out excessive amounts of hormones.

The other tests he ordered (mentioned but not detailed in your post), I'm willing to bet are "thyroid antibodies" ones, to see if the cause of your hyperthyroidism is autoimmune (Graves' disease). The antibodies he ordered might include the TPO and "TSI", the later mentioned being "Thyroid Stimulating Immunoglobulin" - the ones typically found in Graves' disease. He might also be ordering a test of your T3, which is not listed in your post. T repeat, T3 Uptake doesn't measure the T3 hormone level but measures how well the blood uptakes T3 hormone via available binding globulins."

QUESTION EIGHT

Are Non-Prescription Thyroid Glandular Supplements Available?

Most of the thyroid glandular products have the hormones extracted from them because this is the only way they can legally sell it non-prescription. You might read their ingredients to see if this is the case. Also, if it contains iodine, this will not successfully convert into thyroid hormone without your gland present to complete the conversion process (if it is diseased or has been removed). This means that iodine could possibly build in your system over time (not a certainty but a possibility) and this can cause a degree of iodine-toxicity if it goes too high (a hyperthyroid state). On the other hand, if you monitor the effects of the supplement closely and ask your doctor for copies of your repeat blood tests of thyroid hormone levels, this too can help tell you if the supplement is interfering with your hormone replacement therapy (if being administered) or if it is actually aiding it. I'm a believer in natural supplements but in some cases when you require hormone replacement for which there is no substitute, they can hinder the needed, prescription therapy.

No two cases are exactly the same and each patient can be different in this respect, so using the safeguards I mention above (monitoring) can help determine if the supplement is helping or hindering.

QUESTION NINE

Is Determining the Cause of Hypothyroidism Important?

According to medical research, some cases of Hashimoto's thyroiditis (common autoimmune cause of hypothyroidism) do not present with positive antibodies tests but will be detected by Fine Needle Aspiration (thyroid tissue biopsy). Here's the title of one source that mentions this:

"Hashimoto's thyroiditis: fine-needle aspirations of 50 asymptomatic cases." (look for the article on the "PubMed" website).

Viral thyroiditis and sub acute usually present with hyperthyroidism (overactive) and resolve within a few weeks and are not followed by hypothyroidism.

Analysis of a thyroid tissue sample would be differentiated by a reviewing specialist.

Supplements that contain high levels of iodine have been shown to contribute to thyroid autoimmunity resulting in either Grave's disease (autoimmune hyperthyroidism) or Hashimoto's thyroiditis in some people who take them.

If the cause is not within the gland itself - "primary", it can be a "secondary cause". Since there are many possible causes, including secondary ones such as other disease processes going on in the body, age-related (if elderly), thyroid regulating brain gland problems (Central Hypothyroidism), etc..., it may take considerable testing and a process of elimination to find a definitive cause.

Many doctors aren't too concerned about "cause" they simply treat the under active thyroid and if treatment improves it, they call it good. Most patients do however want to know the cause if at all possible (some doctors do too), simply to know what's going on in their bodies. I recently heard from a man, who wrote me in regard to developing hypothyroidism after he had been taking an herbal supplement.

Eighty-Seven Thyroid Disease Questions Answered!

He felt the supplement triggered a case of thyroiditis in his thyroid gland. It is possible that the supplement the man had been taking was causing the hypothyroidism and stopping the herbal might have corrected it. It's hard to imagine that it would have caused permanent damage unless thyroid autoimmunity resulted from it or there was some other agent in it that caused damage to the gland. People vary in their tolerance to herbal supplements, so anything is possible.

In my opinion as a layperson - non medical professional, the T4 and T3 hormone levels should be blood tested to see if only the T3 is lowering in new cases of hypothyroidism that have no cause determined for them. This can happen with "low T3 syndromes" like Wilson's Temperature Syndrome and Euthyroid Sick Syndrome and in cardiac disease patients.

QUESTION TEN

Is Vitamin D Deficiency and Thyroid Autoimmunity Connected?

Vitamin D deficiency has been found in medical research to cause immune system problems. There have been studies showing that it places people with both deficiency (blood-level readings of 20 ng/mL and below) and insufficiency (blood-level readings of 30 ng/mL and below) at risk for autoimmune disease and other chronic and inflammatory diseases, including those affecting the thyroid gland.

My reason for researching on the D deficiency syndromes, is due to my personally being diagnosed with deficiency (my result was "17 ng/mL"), which I'm currently being treated for. I have Hashimoto's thyroiditis caused hypothyroidism and I now have yet another possible cause of mine, being vitamin D deficiency.

Autoimmune thyroiditis very rarely goes into remission or I should say rarely reverses but is usually life-long and replacing low vitamin D levels is very important but will not cure the disease, if it is already present.

Eighty-Seven Thyroid Disease Questions Answered!

So far no treatments have been found to cure autoimmunity of any kind although patients with Graves' disease can see hyperthyroidism permanently resolved with thyroid removal or ablation with radioactive iodine. They do afterward have to be treated permanently with thyroid hormone replacement.

One thing that does help reduce thyroid antibodies (the immune cells that cause the disease) according to med-research, is supplementing with selenium at the recommended dose on the label. Other than this way to reduce it to some degree, there's no cure for the thyroid autoimmunity itself. I wish there were because I would certainly get it administered for mine, if there were. Some sources I went to, to search about Drisdol (my prescribed treatment for D-deficiency) state that it's a "D2" replacement vitamin. I looked at my prescription bottle and it says Generic for: DRISDOL . It also states on the label: "50,000UNT" (the mega-dose size). The manufacturer is shown as: "BRENC" (apparently an abbreviation for the company that makes it). Some sources state that deficiency needs to be treated with "D3" rather than D2 for better improvement.

I'm going to be retested on my 25(OH)D level in a couple months (a name for D levels in the body) and at regular intervals of about once a year, thereafter. If I remember correctly the blood test shows both D2 and D3 levels (I always get copies of all labs I have done). While my original deficiency reading was "17" as mentioned previously, even a level of 30 is considered "insufficiency" and I believe they like to see the level increased to at least 50 or above.

If this Vitamin D brand doesn't get my levels corrected properly, as reflected in follow-up blood retests, I will definitely ask for a change to D3 supplementation.

QUESTION ELEVEN

Increased Anxiety Symptoms with Hypothyroid Treatment, Following RAI?

This article is my response to a thyroid patient who underwent Radio Active Iodine destruction of their thyroid gland (RAI Ablation) and upon becoming hypothyroid following; they were started on replacement hormone therapy.

Eighty-Seven Thyroid Disease Questions Answered!

31

The new hormone dose was causing some bodily adjustment symptoms of anxiety and following was my response to them in regard to this. ---

"I'm sorry to hear you are struggling with the anxiety. I've been there and now how terribly unpleasant it can be! Mine did improve greatly and I believe yours will too, over time. It's hard to be patient when you feel miserable but I would encourage you, that with your ongoing treatment and blood retests, your doctor will know how to adjust your replacement dose of thyroid hormone. Once you are better leveled-out, which can take some time, following radioactive iodine treatment (the thyroid ablation you mentioned having), you'll see the anxiety symptoms improve.

It's a strange phenomenon because it can actually cause hypothyroid therapy to induce even more anxiety at first but once you are on a proper dose of prescribed hormone, you should see the anxiety symptoms improve after a few months (maybe as little as 8 weeks). When I say proper dose, many reputable thyroid specialists believe the TSH level needs to be suppressed down to "1.0" for patients to see optimal symptom improvement.

Average lab normal ranges are from "0.5 to 5.0".

In my case, it took a few months after I was on proper thyroid dose to see my anxiety symptoms improve significantly. Mine did actually increase for a while, especially during the first few weeks on my initial dose."

QUESTION TWELVE

Can Anxiety Symptoms Occur with Taking a Thyroid Hormone Dose?

This article was my response to a hypothyroid patient who wrote me in regard to experiencing anxiety symptoms while adjusting to a new dose of replacement hormone therapy (Note: This Q&A was similar to that of the previous chapter but RAI was not involved). ---

"I can relate to what you are going through. The first doctor, who treated me, placed me on a full replacement dose of thyroid hormone, immediately (Synthroid), when.

Most doctors like to start at a lower dose and build it up to full-replacement. It kicked-in very strong anxiety symptoms that literally made me pace a circle in my living room because my resting heart rate went up to about 150 and I was hyperventilating. Once I was on a stable, correct dose for about two months, the anxiety resolved for the most part.

Yes, both too low a dose and too high a dose can cause anxiety symptoms. A low dose causes your body to try compensating for lack of thyroid hormone by increasing adrenaline, which is the same thing that happens to hypoglycemic people when their blood sugar/glucose goes too low. A dose that's too high causes anxiety for obvious reasons, because the metabolism is being spiked too much, too quickly.

Thyroid hormone therapy is a delicate balance but some doctors don't approach it that way and think any reading that's within normal values is good. The fact is however, that some patients need a sustained optimized level of hormone in their body. It could be that given a few more weeks, your current dose will adjust better in your body because it usually takes 8-weeks or so for this to happen.

Eighty-Seven Thyroid Disease Questions Answered!

I will have to say that I'm surprised your doctor does not see the importance in retesting your blood level to monitor the new dose and if he still doesn't agree to do so within a few more weeks, I would find a doctor who is willing to do so. If you're still walking around with an imbalanced thyroid level, this needs to be determined or it needs to be confirmed that the level is good. Blood levels are the most accurate way to know if you have good levels or need an adjustment to them, to regain a euthroid state (normalized)."

QUESTION THIRTEEN

What do Positive Thyroid Antibodies Mean?

The positive thyroid antibodies blood test means you have autoimmune thyroid disease. Your doctor will likely do further testing, if not already done, to determine if you have Hashimoto's thyroiditis, which causes hypothyroidism (under active), or if you have Graves' disease, which causes hyperthyroidism (overactive).

This will depend on what a thyroid panel shows - whether your thyroid hormones are decreasing or increasing as a result of the antibodies attacking/attaching to your thyroid gland. You didn't mention which type antibodies were found positive but if it was the TPO or TG ones, this would point to Hashimoto's if your thyroid hormones (T4 and T3) are also low and/or if your TSH is found to be high (elevated). The opposite will be true of these (low TSH and high thyroid hormones), if Graves' disease is the case.

First Hashimoto's can be diagnosed no matter how long you've been on thyroid hormone. They detect it via the "anti-TPO" and "anti-TG" antibodies tests and I would bet strongly that yours would return positive on either or both. Ask your doctor to order these because it will only take him a stroke of the pen to do so. Some believe the 'cause' of hypothyroidism isn't important but I feel a patient has a right to know if it is autoimmune (hashi's disease or Grave's) because autoimmune diseases place a person at slightly higher risk for other metabolic and autoimmune diseases, like diabetes and rheumatoid arthritis.

As per your question as to what type of doctor I prefer for my own health provider needs -- an Osteopath (D.O.) is actually my preferred Dr. because they believe in a degree of natural supplements, in-balance but do not go as far with them as do naturopaths (Note: there is no substitute when prescribed thyroid hormone is needed). D.O. physicians also require more education than do regular MDs/GPs and they can be just as board certified as any other MD and can deliver babies, perform surgeries and prescribe medications.

QUESTION FOURTEEN

Any Medical Research Available on Anxiety and Thyroid Disease?

Lots of medical research states that autoimmune thyroiditis can cause anxiety symptoms and even anxiety disorders in some patients.

Following are some quotes in regard to this:

- - -

" In a study of patients with Hashimoto's thyroiditis, anxiety was a prominent initial symptom at the time that the condition was diagnosed." (Richard Hall MD PhD - Johns Hopkins) - LINK> http://www.drrichardhall.com/anxiety.htm

"The study seems to suggest that individuals in the community with thyroid autoimmunity may be at high risk for mood and anxiety disorders. The psychiatric disorders and the autoimmune reaction seem to be rooted in a same (and not easily correctable) aberrancy in the immuno-endocrine system." (U.S. NIH) - LINK> PubMed.com

"We have found that sub clinical thyroid dysfunction increases the anxiety of patients whether hyperthyroid or hypothyroid." (U.S. NIH) - LINK> PubMed.com

These studies quoted above, are not even in regard to yet another condition that can occur with thyroiditis called "Hashitoxicosis" (intermittent or temporary hyperthyroidism), which can occur in some Hashimoto's patients, before progressive hypothyroidism sets-in.

Eighty-Seven Thyroid Disease Questions Answered!

"Hashitoxicosis is a transient hyperthyroidism caused by inflammation associated with Hashimoto's thyroiditis disturbing the thyroid follicles, resulting in excess release of thyroid hormone." LINK> Hashitoxicosis - Wikipedia, the free encyclopedia

These sources make it very clear that anxiety can occur with autoimmune thyroiditis.

QUESTION FIFTEEN

Are There Side-Effects Adjusting to a New Thyroid Hormone Dose?

Thyroid hormone replacement takes about eights weeks for a new dose to fully adjust in the body and to begin doing its job. Treatment can take longer however, depending on how many dose-adjustments are needed to get you to adequate/optimal levels. Many patients need one or two adjustments because Dr.s often start at a low dose and increase it upward which is called "titrating the dose". You should see more symptom-resolution as more weeks go by.

Eighty-Seven Thyroid Disease Questions Answered!

All types/brands of prescribed thyroid hormone are designed to take over the thyroid gland's production, which is inadequate when hypothyroidism is present. As the hormone comes in from outside of the body, the pituitary gland (in the brain) senses the increase in the blood stream and sends less TSH to the thyroid gland (Thyroid Stimulating Hormone). For some hypothyroid patients, they will experience a break-even point, before improvement from increasing thyroid hormone levels begins to occur.

Also: Many medical research articles also attribute hypothyroid symptoms to the "thyroid autoimmunity" aspect of thyroid disease, rather than just to the abnormal or fluctuating thyroid hormone levels but some doctors aren't aware of this fact.

SECTION TWO: Questions and Answers SIXTEEN through THIRTY

QUESTION SIXTEEN

Is there a Need for Synthetic and Natural Thyroid Hormone?

I've read articles in regard to how, in the early days of treating hypothyroid patients, they fed them raw animal thyroid glands. The patients usually did very well on this strange method of treatment. Just the fact that thyrotoxicity (treatment-induced hyperthyroidism) happens with taking too high a dose of thyroid hormone replacement (patients testify to this happening today), is why safeguards are in place for present-day treatments. Is the system perfect? As you and I know, of course not. When patients don't respond favorably to the standard treatment, doctors need to look at every single area of the hormone replacement to see if it can be tweaked (adjusted for improvement) even more. Every avenue should be explored for improving a patient's treatment, including exceeding the maximum dose to some degree (as agreed between Dr. and patient, as reflected on blood retest levels).

Only then, should other causes for unresolved hypothyroid symptoms be looked into.

I am one of those patients who didn't do well on Synthroid, synthetic T-4 only medication and I was switched to Armour brand – natural T4 and T3 combination and began doing significantly better. My mother however has been on Synthroid for many years now and has done very well, with no need for switching her brand. When I mentioned Armour to her several times, asking if she thought she might do even better, she refused to inquire with her doctor about it because of feeling so well on the Synthroid and she didn't want to upset the applecart so to speak (why try fixing something that's not broken?).

I have read that some people actually have the opposite effect happen to them - they have bad reaction to Armour and are switched back to a synthetic brand (either T4 only or a combo T3 and T4). Some people for example, are allergic to porcine products, pork etc.... If Armour (made from pig thyroid glands) was the only brand available, what would happen to these hypothyroid people needing treatment?

Is Armour superior in treating hypothyroidism? For some people it absolutely is superior and extremely-so, in some cases. This may actually be true in a majority of cases but synthetic still needs to be available for people who need another option, including those who cannot take the brand due to their religious affiliation, requiring kosher observance (consuming no pig by-products) or their allergy to porcine products.

A patient's excitement and pro-activeness in advocating for a particular thyroid hormone brand, is a good thing and may someday contribute to causing reform of those things in regard to hypothyroid treatments that aren't good (i.e. treating according to lab ranges only, with no consideration for unresolved symptoms). This is true of those who advocate for synthetic brands as well.

QUESTION SEVENTEEN

What's the Difference between Optimal versus Over-treated Hypothyroidism?

I am on 150mg (2.5 -grains) of Armour brand - thyroid hormone replacement therapy. I was first placed on Synthroid three years previous to my Armour dosing and my Dr. switched me due to concern I was one of those patients who has problems with 'T-4 to T-3 conversion' (also called 'impaired conversion'). As far as my having been on the dose I describe in another article, that suppressed my TSH to 0.006 (far below normal), I was on that dose for several months, which placed me at risk for becoming toxic on the thyroid hormone (TSH goes lower as thyroid hormones rise in the body). My intermittent joint and fatigue symptoms did not improve but the fatigue worsened dramatically after I had been on the higher dose for about three months. As far as heart problems at hyperthyroid levels (the "hyperthyroid" term is used interchangeably with hormone-toxicity) and the many other serious problems it can cause, I'll give you a first hand example of what hyperthyroidism, regardless of cause, can do to a person. ---

Eighty-Seven Thyroid Disease Questions Answered!

My Uncle had Graves Disease and became hyperthyroid as a result. It was not treated for too long of a period and in addition to dramatic weight loss, he developed a heart aneurism, needing corrected by surgery. He also experienced a stroke from delayed treatment of the hyperthyroidism. The reason Dr.s equate thyroid hormone toxicity (also called thyrotoxicosis), with hyperthyroidism, is because it can have identically the same effects on a person.

Treatment-individuality of patients on hypothyroid therapy needs considered, I agree, which is why symptomatic treatment, without TSH testing/monitoring cannot be safe for every patient. One reason is because with some people, the line between thyrotoxicosis (over-treatment) and being asymptomatic can be a very fine/thin line. Also, my unresolved symptoms, that I attempted to resolve by increasing my thyroid hormone dose, were almost certainly not thyroid related (I was later found to have 3 vitamin deficiencies). You may remember in Mary Shomon's book "Living Well With Autoimmune Disease", if you have read it, that she states with her thyroid medication dose optimized, she had lingering symptoms and was also diagnosed with co morbid CFS/Fibromyalgia.

Eighty-Seven Thyroid Disease Questions Answered!

She takes low-dose antibiotics to relieve her joint pain and on her Thyroid-Info website she stated in an article, that at one time she went off the antibiotics and the joint pain/fatigue returned. I do not know if she still requires an antibiotic or if she was able at some point to discontinue them.

My opinion is that a well treated thyroid condition can still have co morbid conditions existing with it (medical sources state that 25% of patients with thyroid autoimmunity experience other autoimmune diseases). My belief is that there are subtle viral infections, allergies etc... that can cause symptoms as separate entity-illnesses. I for example, have low cortisol levels but not Addison's disease (Adrenal Fatigue). In fact, I had a cortisol test result recently, of "1.7" in a normal range of "3 to 8 ng/mL". Not only does thyroid hormone not treat low adrenal conditions but it can actually lower thr adrenal cortisol hormone even further in people with varied degrees of adrenal insufficiency, which means it is separate issue, needing separate attention. ALL THINGS cannot be linked to thyroid but I certainly believe thyroid patients need to be optimized to the best possible levels on their thyroid hormone dose that also does not place them at risk for over-treatment.

Eighty-Seven Thyroid Disease Questions Answered!

Thyrotoxicosis from over-replacement is a genuine possibility. As far as the question of whether I have actually heard of people going hyperthyroid from over-replacement, the answer is "Yes, I have seen people's testimonials of having this experience, many, many times on thyroid info websites and message boards.

QUESTION EIGHTEEN

Any Opinions on the Thyroid Stimulating Hormone Blood Test Debate?

I would like to express something about the TSH treatment-level debate (Thyroid Stimulating Hormone – blood tests). First let me say I sometimes -- for lack of a better term, "play dumb" when I inquire about a subject on thyroid patient discussion-forums, so that I get unprompted opinions and so that I'm not leading an answer I might get, in the direction I want it to go. When I tell someone I agree with them, I may be speaking about a specific, not a blanket agreement on everything.

Eighty-Seven Thyroid Disease Questions Answered!

Second, I want to admit, that the suggestion about suppressing TSH (it elevates with hypothyroidism) to almost undetectable levels before some patients experience symptomatic relief, led me to finally experiment in this area, with my own medication, which I strongly and emphatically DISCOURAGE anyone from doing. I did-so because of desperation for symptom relief, including ongoing joint pain flares and severe fatigue spells. I do some contract work requiring a lot of physical stamina and I need a certain amount of wellness, to keep going. I very slowly increased my thyroid hormone medication, above that recommended by my Dr., until my TSH was almost undetectable. I did not have any hyper/toxicity symptoms from this but I experienced a severe, bone numbing fatigue, which means I likely was at the edge of dangerous reactions to the dose. My symptoms did not improve. I am now at the dose-level originally recommended by my Dr., with a TSH between 0.5 to 1.0.

My opinion is that "certain" people have a pituitary response (the gland that sends out TSH in response to thyroid hormone levels) that is sluggish but not actually at the "hypopituitarism" level (under-functioning pituitary gland).

Eighty-Seven Thyroid Disease Questions Answered!

Their Free T-3 and other levels can be upper, but not top-normal and their TSH will already be suppressed to near undetectable level. The problem is - how can a Dr. assume someone is in this category, when the majority of people are not? This is why a standard is set that covers the majority of people treated for hypothyroidism. Most Endocrinologists and thyroid specialists, even the AACE (American Association of Clinical Endocrinologists), recommends a treatment TSH level below 3.0, so the goal of 0.5 to 1.0, is even more optimal. To narrow it even further, is simply too risky for the majority of people. Hyper-toxicity (thyrotoxicity) from over-treatment (hyperthyroidism induced by too high a dose) can actually be life-threatening and no-one should want to see that risk taken on wide scales but only with those individuals who apparently have a slight pituitary abnormality and need a little more attention with maximum dosing. These people need repeat testing of their other hormone levels besides TSH. I think what happens is that someone who does obtain optimal symptom relief by symptomatic adjustment of their thyroid hormone dose, rather than by using the in-range cautions, believes their experience proves this success goes for everyone who might attempt this and they are understandably very excited about it.

In reality, the majority of people need a TSH level at the low-normal cut-off range or they can be at very serious risk for things like heart arrhythmia problems and chronic bone loss (osteoporosis).

QUESTION NINTEEN

Does Polyglandular Autoimmune Disease Occur in Thyroid Patients?

There are complications that can off-spring, so-to-speak from autoimmune thyroid disease (Hashimoto's thyroiditis). Diabetes is one of them but patients are practically never informed about this. I know this from corresponding with 100s of fellow patients over the years, since 2003. Some of the diseases that can develop in people with autoimmune hypothyroidism are "Polyglandular Autoimmune Diseases" and there are two categories of these. One type is a combination of Hashimoto's and Addison's disease (adrenal insufficiency) and they also refer to this one as "Schmidt's Syndrome" or "PGA I".

The other is a combination of several diseases such as Hashimoto's with adult onset diabetes (type II), adrenal insufficiency and hypo-parathyroid disease - a dysfunction in the endocrine glands that regulate calcium levels in the body. When these glands become either hyper-functioning (high) or hypo-functioning (low), they can cause symptoms similar to hypothyroidism. This other type of polyglandular problem affecting several glands in the body is referred-to as "PGA II".

Dizziness upon standing (Orthostatic Hypotension) can be a major symptom of low adrenal function, especially when you experience it severely enough to actually pass out from episodes of it (syncope). They usually check your cortisol (cortical) levels and for adrenal antibodies, to rule out or diagnose the presence of adrenal dysfunction/disease. They may also test to see how well the adrenals respond to being stimulated, via the "ACTH Stimulation Test". The other co morbid disorders that can occur with autoimmune thyroiditis, are detected via testing for imbalances in these other endocrine glands, if they suspect that problems have developed in them.

QUESTION TWENTY

Are There 'Thyroid Removal' Options for Hashimoto's Thyroiditis?

From what I have read on many medical sources, many people are found to have Hashimoto's Disease, even when their thyroid hormones are all within normal-range. I'm sure you know this but for sake of those who might not and are reading this, Hashimoto's is an autoimmune disease with no cure and it causes hypothyroidism at different rates of progression. Some people have it for many years before having symptoms. Other people are discovered having it, along with a goiter (thyroid swelling) being the only initial, physical symptom. Other medical information I have read states that the autoimmune attack that causes this common form of thyroiditis causes symptoms in some patients even before hypothyroidism sets-in but the majority of doctors do not recognize this fact. Be prepared that if you suggest treatment be started for you, due to confirmed Hashimoto's but normal thyroid hormones (unless you have a more informed doctor), that he/she will likely tell you, you're having emotional problems not related to your thyroid disease.

After all, "your other labs (apart from positive antibodies) are within normal range".

I hate to say it but I am so glad my TSH and T-3 Uptake were both out of range, indicating hypothyroidism, on my very first blood tests. I didn't have antibodies checked until 2-years later because the doctor I was seeing wouldn't order them for me. When I did have the tests performed, both my TG and TPO ABs were elevated. I had terrible anxiety symptoms, mixed with depression for MONTHS before getting that first test and even though I told my doctor at that time that I felt it was my thyroid causing symptoms, she prescribed an anti-depressant, Xanax (anti-anxiety drug) and a beta-blocker to treat my symptoms, rather than testing me for treatable thyroid hormone imbalances. My symptoms worsened as a result.

When I finally demanded that first blood test, they failed to notify me regarding results. More than a month later, I called the Doctor's office, asking "where's my test result?". They said: "Sorry it must have gotten lost for a while but there is nothing on the report indicating anything needing treatment." I then called the lab itself and asked for a copy, which they were able to provide, via my signing a release.

I had two abnormal readings on the thyroid panel (High TSH and Low T-3 Uptake), plus elevated cholesterol (another sign of hypothyroidism). I took the results to a new doctor and he placed me on thyroid hormone replacement medication, although he did say "It's only a sub-clinical case of hypothyroidism". Since then, I have required four dose increases of my hormone drug and may have more to come in the future (I'm now on 150mg - Armour).

I would certainly research about thyroidectomy or oblation (RAI killing off or surgical removal of the thyroid) before going through with one of these procedures for your Hashimoto's thyroiditis. It is usually restricted to cases of Graves' disease – hyperthyroidism. You will basically have the same result letting your gland die out gradually through the antibodies process over time. You will need full thyroid hormone replacement therapy, once it is removed following the procedures I have mentioned. I don't know if all people who undergo thyroid removal have to have dose adjustments or not or if some are given a full replacement dose that is started and maintained, with little or no adjustment needed (this likely varies with each patient).

Eighty-Seven Thyroid Disease Questions Answered!

I would research about all possible post-effects of the ablation procedure before I would have it done but I also wonder if a Dr. would even seriously consider it, without your lab ranges being more outside of normal values or without severe thyroid pain occurring in your case. I believe Hashimoto's patients can have fluctuating symptoms also due to life events (stressors) and the same is true of Graves'-hyperthyroidism. The reason I believe this is because people with proper functioning thyroids, will have it adjust automatically to extra mental stressors and extra physical activity, that obviously places more demand on their bodies for increased thyroid hormone levels. With hypothyroid patients, we are on a set-dose of replacement hormone, so that we are operating on the same amount no matter what extra demands are placed on our bodies due to emotional/physical stress, illnesses, etc...., which is why adequate replacement dose-levels are so important.

Again, I would suggest researching your treatment options and discuss them fully with your doctor, including asking about risks involved, should you be offered the option of ablation (radioactive thyroid destruction) or removal of your gland, surgically.

QUESTION TWENTY-ONE

Any Comments on Diagnosing and Treating Autoimmune Hyperthyroidism?

Derived from a forum post I wrote in 2005. ---

When I mentioned "borderline" (in reply to your post) I only meant on the TSH reading you were bordering on being flagged low. Borderline just means right on the edge of being abnormal (TSH drops low with hyperthyroid conditions). As far as the condition itself that you might have, causing your over-active thyroid, only complete testing can reveal if it's full blown Grave's disease (autoimmune hyperthyroidism) or if it is just entering that phase of abnormal for some other reason. You are right about antibodies being the test to see if the hyperthyroidism is autoimmune or not because there are secondary causes of hyperthyroidism, such as a pituitary gland that puts out too much TSH, due to a tumor within it (rare) etc...however, your TSH is low, so that probably rules out the pituitary as your cause of <u>overactive</u> thyroid.

If you have elevated antibodies along with hyperthyroidism (especially the "TSI" ABs), that pretty much reveals the cause right there, as being "Grave's Autoimmune Hyperthyroidism". Blood tests will reveal if it's autoimmune and there's also the possibility of either or both a goiter and nodules (overall swelling and small tumors in the gland) being present. Goiter is thyroid swelling, while nodules are small growths, common in both hypothyroid and hyperthyroid patients, with autoimmunity as the cause. Most nodules are benign but some can be malignant and others can cause extra release of thyroid hormones (hot nodules).

Sometimes it's good to get a second opinion. I did this back when I was struggling with Hashimoto's Disease (autoimmune hypothyroidism), trying to get diagnosed and coincidentally, it was the thyroid antibodies test that actually finally told me what was causing my hypothyroidism. I too got second opinions in my case and never told my regular doctor because I felt it was none of his business unless I completely switched to a new doctor and needed my medical records transferred.

Your current Doctor seemed to think the only treatment was to remove or ablate (destroy via radioactive iodine), part of the gland but that is usually only done, in milder cases of hyperthyroidism, if medications don't control symptoms. Do you have high blood pressure or tachycardia (rapid heart beat)? If you do, it is strange that she isn't concerned about it as a complication of your abnormal increase in metabolism. Maybe your symptoms are mild enough, that she doesn't want to consider these other medications at this point but your mention of panic attacks made me think your vital signs might be operating very high. Xanax might calm down your nerves but I'm not sure it would help with the hypertension and high heart rate (tachycardia). Your case definitely needs investigated further and followed-up on and you might consider a 'second opinion' by a qualified thyroid specialist or endocrinologist.

QUESTION TWENTY-TWO

Should Doctors Consider Hypothyroidism Symptoms versus Lab Results Only?

It's always disappointing, hearing about a Dr. that won't treat a patient who has severe symptoms of under active thyroid, just because their lab ranges aren't out of range enough yet. I believe you said antibodies were already found to be positive in your case (per your post). That means your thyroid hormone "receptors" can be blocked by the antibodies, causing hypothyroid symptoms, even with hormone levels in normal range, according to some medical websites. Also, the antibodies can cause development of goiter and/or thyroid nodules (tumors – usually benign) and thyroid replacement medication can halt this or reduce already existing ones in the gland.

Some Dr.s who treat hypothyroidism are "lab-range only" ones and others look at these other issues listed above and other types of symptom-manifestations to determine the timing of starting a patient on treatment.

Some Dr.s claim it is their concern over making a patient go "HYPERthyroid" if they treat too early and that this can cause osteoporosis and heart arrhythmias however, why can't they reassure against this through follow-up blood testing, just like with other patients on treatment for hypothyroidism? Websites I've researched claim that the osteoporosis possibility has been completely blown out of proportion and does not occur easily, unless a patient is severely over-treated for long periods of time. As far as heart arrhythmias go, if they begin to occur, a Dr. might simply reduce the dosage slightly, to alleviate them.

You might consider a second opinion if a doctor is reluctant to treat mild but symptomatic hypothyroidism but make sure you take all lab results with you and always get copies of all labs each time tests are completed.

I personally would never use herbal methods to treat a thyroid disorder. I believe people who do, are playing with fire! You need Dr. Supervision and blood testing follow-ups for hypothyroidism to be treated properly.

I get very passionate about bad Dr. Treatment but I have EVERY CONFIDENCE in the good ones out there, of which **there are many**. While there are plenty of good, quality physicians, the trick is in finding them.

In regard to the antibodies present in most cases of hypothyroidism (Hashimoto's disease) , there is no cure for them and they cause a disease process in the thyroid gland that is most often life-long. They have to run their course, although thyroid hormone replacement medication may significantly lower the antibodies levels over time in some patients. SO THERE IS another positive reason for starting thyroid replacement medication in patients with the autoimmune type disease in their thyroid glands.

The antibodies will keep attacking until there's no more living thyroid tissue left to attack and so a patient who is not yet at a level of hypothyroidism that requires treatment, will reach that level at some point -- some sooner than others.

QUESTION TWENTY-THREE

Can Antibiotics Aggravate Thyroid Autoimmunity?

Antibodies from the immune system are natural and produced by the body and are specific toward the invader they need to attack. Its amazing how the body can make these toward whatever needs eradicated, such as allergens and bacteria's we are exposed to. Antibiotics on the other hand are micro-organisms produced by man, for administering to people with infections caused by bacteria but they are ineffective against viruses.

Could antibiotics attack antibodies that go against one of our organs? This I don't know, does anyone else out there have an answer for this? There is supposedly an antibiotic that a select few people have taken and it cured their Hashimoto's thyroiditis but I will not believe this until I see it announced on reputable medical sources (it would be nice though).

I really don't believe there is any chance of antibiotics increasing thyroid antibodies, one they are administered to someone to treat an infection.

They are actually two different things and I believe they would continue to do their separate jobs, although we don't like the job the thyroid antibodies are doing in cases of autoimmunity in the gland (disease process).

I don't think there is any danger at all in people with thyroid autoimmunity taking antibiotics and I'm sure Hashimoto's patients are placed on these type drugs as often as anyone else. You might however, want to tell a Dr. or Dentist that you have Hashimoto's, when they suggest antibiotics or any other medication, just as a precaution, to see if they believe there could be any adverse interactions (contraindications).

QUESTION TWENTY-FOUR

Does Thyroid Disease Cause Emotional Symptoms?

This article is derived from a forum post I wrote in 2005. ---

"There is a very definite problem with doctors telling patients their emotional problems are not due to their thyroid disorders, when the patient knows for a fact that it is. They believe a person only attributes the emotional issues to thyroid because they don't want to admit having an emotional problem. EVERYONE has a certain degree of anxiety and depression, at times, or they are not human because these are natural emotions but thyroid disorder people develop more problematic type emotional problems and they know for a fact it came with development of their thyroid condition. The second Dr. I went to after I was diagnosed hypothyroid, I asked; "Can hypothyroidism cause anxiety & depression"? He replied; "No, only tiredness." After he told me this, I got online and went to website-after-website by reputable medical sources and every one of them listed "depression" as one of the most common symptoms of hypothyroidism.

Eighty-Seven Thyroid Disease Questions Answered!

Many of them included "anxiety" as a symptom as well. Other websites, containing lots of personal stories by hypothyroid patients, commonly had them mentioning anxiety along with the depression that was caused by their thyroid condition.

Why do some doctors want to see the emotional symptoms as not being related to the thyroid condition, especially when they are not completely relieved by treatment? Who knows for sure but I do know they are relentlessly pushed by pharmaceutical companies, to mass-prescribe antidepressants and doctors themselves often admit this (I heard one refer to this recently on a radio program).

If a thyroid patient does not have adequate dose of thyroid medication and this causes symptoms to linger, why not let an optimized dose be reached and given a chance to relieve symptoms before an antidepressant is prescribed? This has always been my question in light of the increasing frequency of antidepressant prescribing to hypothyroid patients who are inadequately treated on thyroid hormone. If a thyroid patient complains that their symptoms haven't been relieved as expected, the first thing a Dr. should do is check to see if they need a dosage increase of their hormone replacement therapy.

Hashimoto's patients commonly develop a need for dose increases due to the thyroid gland progressively dying-out (atrophy)."

QUESTION TWENTY-FIVE

Is Combining Antidepressants with Hypothyroid Therapy Okay?

I was placed on an antidepressant when I went to a Doctor feeling ill and I finally weaned slowly off of it when I requested my own blood lab tests and it was found that I had autoimmune hypothyroidism.

Let me say that I believe antidepressants can be very helpful to people and I personally know people who are on them and doing great. The reason I personally got off of them is because my root problem was not emotionally caused, it was thyroid disease caused. I wanted treatment for it before I considered an antidepressant, so that I would not confuse thyroid symptoms with the drug side effects.

Some of the antidepressant side effects are; "fatigue, lightheadedness, dizziness, sexual dysfunction, nervousness, tremor", etc.... -- the same as are listed for thyroid hormone imbalances.

PLEASE UNDERSTAND, I am not suggesting that anyone quit taking the antidepressant they are prescribed, what I am saying is that If you find through lab testing that you have hypothyroidism, you need to get treatment for it, in addition to the antidepressant because an untreated thyroid disorder can be worsened with antidepressant treatment alone. SSRI antidepressants can lower thyroid hormones even further, when one has autoimmune hypothyroidism, according to research I have read, so they can affect the need for dose adjustments in thyroid hormone treated patients. Many medical sites state this but one study I can refer to in particular is one from Sept., 2004, conducted by "UCLA School of Medicine, Dept of Endocrinology" THEIR CONCLUSION: "With Antidepressant treatment, the most common change in thyroid hormones is a DECREASE in T-4 and Free T-4." That study tells me, if you have hypothyroidism, an antidepressant can potentially make it worse if left untreated and unmonitored.

QUESTION TWENTY-SIX

Is There Importance in a Qualified Thyroid Doctor?

I know there are top-notch thyroid doctors out there but they are becoming rare. If you can get in to see a specialist for thyroid disorders, I would certainly consider it.

Dr.s sometimes use the psychosomatic (emotional) explanation for unrelieved symptoms of treated thyroid disorder, when it is a difficult case. This of course is possible with any patient and any disorder but I personally do not believe it is the case with as many patients as they seem to believe it occurs in. I say this because I personally know people who were under-treated for their thyroid disorders plus have read testimonies of hundreds of others, who were told their symptoms were mood-related or imagined. How can this many people be having imagined or emotionally caused symptoms? Common sense tells me it is related to their thyroid disorders and they need more specialized care. My last two doctors were Endocrinologists and they still gave me strange advice, so you need to check references etc... to choose a good one that is genuinely qualified in thyroid treatments.

Examples of things I was told by my Endo-doctors: "Your TSH is on the edge of high-normal (elevates with hypothyroid and the goal of treatment is suppress it) but since it is within the reference range, your symptoms cannot be thyroid related" and: "You have Autoimmune Hypothyroidism but is probably only temporary." (actually it is lifelong in the vast majority of cases)... And: "It is extremely rare to have adrenal insufficiency or another autoimmune disease with Hashimoto's thyroiditis (actually, some medical sources state that 25% of patients develop co morbid health disorders, much of it being other autoimmune diseases)."

The fact is, that the TSH has to be low-normal, not high-normal, for a hypothyroid patient to feel better on thyroid hormone replacement. ALSO, Hashimoto's requires life-long treatment with hormone replacement and people who have experienced remission of the disease are the ones who are "extremely rare". ALSO, One in four (25%) of Hashimoto's patients develop other related disorders as referred above. The above is why I say you might need a second opinion from a qualified specialist, in case you were misdiagnosed or are not getting optimal treatment.

Eighty-Seven Thyroid Disease Questions Answered!

Under-treatment for thyroid patients is way too common and will take people like us to help make a difference, through 'patient advocacy' (sharing our experiences and self-educating, in order to share your knowledge with other patients). I sometimes wonder if doctors are required to update their knowledge in thyroid treatment protocols, since so many new things have been learned over the past several years. If not, we really can't place full blame on the doctors who are not being updated via available avenues. Maybe new requirements for updates to Doctors should be enforced, so that inadequate treatment cases can be reduced.

QUESTION TWENTY-SEVEN

Is There Varied Effectiveness of Antidepressants in Thyroid Patients?

From a forum post I made in 2005. ---

"If I remember right, I think you said on a past post (my comments are directed toward another forum member), that you had a high TSH on your blood tests.

Eighty-Seven Thyroid Disease Questions Answered!

From what I understand Grave's disease never causes an elevated TSH but a suppressed (low) one. Hashimoto's patients do have hyperthyroid, Grave's type symptoms commonly, early into their Hashimoto's disease. I know I did for a good while and at first I thought it was just severe anxiety. A doctor placed me on Paxil for a few months (an SSRI Antidepressant), a few years ago but for me personally, I couldn't stand the side effects of the drug. I got really trembly and weak in my body (I already suffered from some of this but it became worse with the antidepressant). I also had electric "zap" type sensations that went from my head, all the way down to my toes. It also affected my libido (sex drive), causing a significant drop in it.

Some people may do well on these type drugs but I didn't (other patients attest to this as well). It took quit a few weeks for me to completely feel free of the lingering build-up of the antidepressant in my system, when I weaned off the drug very slowly with my doctor's help. Please don't let this be a discouragement to anyone out there because as I said, some people may benefit a great deal from SSRI-Antidepressants but I am one patient who didn't. A trial of the drug is needed, to determine its benefits or side effect draw backs).

Eighty-Seven Thyroid Disease Questions Answered!

I'm glad you SLOWLY came off the antidepressant, because some people stop them abruptly (bad idea) and for some reason, most Dr.s don't warn about this or tell patients about the side-effects and severe withdrawal symptoms from not gradually tapering off of an antidepressant of any kind.

Your hyperthyroid symptoms should improve over time and your hypothyroid symptoms as well but it takes a lot of patience as you better adjust and receive any necessary dose-adjustments."

QUESTION TWENTY-EIGHT

Do Hyperthyroid Symptoms occur from Hypothyroid Therapy?

ALL thyroid medications have the same potential to cause heart arrhythmias and this is usually a matter of taking too much of any of them, that can result in this (the same warning on all of them applies). I take "Armour Thyroid" brand but I was first placed on Synthroid. I didn't have arrhythmias but I had HYPER-thyroid type symptoms when I first started Synthroid.

Eighty-Seven Thyroid Disease Questions Answered!

When I was switched to Armour, I never once had these symptoms.

I've read that some people are more sensitive to the Armour brand (natural T4 and T3) than to the Synthroid (synthetic T4). I believe this is because Armour (made from pig/porcine thyroid glands) has both hormones in it and medical researchers say T-3 has more potential to cause hyper type symptoms such as arrhythmias than does "T-4 only" medications. Even your TSH reading of 1.0 (approximate normal range: 0.5 to 4.5) would seem good because they recommend as low as 0.5 for some people with stubborn hypothyroid symptoms. Yes, you can go from hypo to hyper thyroid with autoimmune thyroiditis, early into the disease and many on this forum have attested to this happening to them. I too, early on, had really severe anxiety and waking up during the night in cold sweats etc... Mine finally went to progressive hypothroidism and stayed there but occasionally I do have some anxiety symptoms. Medical websites I've researched say both hypo and hyper thyroid patients can have anxiety as a manifestation of thyroid autoimmunity, regardless of corrected hormone levels.

As far as hyper swings, that then return back to hypo, this is due to the antibodies attack against the thyroid and its response while it is able, in releasing large spurts of hormone in attempt to compensate against damage being done to it. We, in a sense have germ warfare going on in our bodies you might say! You'll see on medical info sites, that Hashimoto's thyroiditis patients commonly have hyper swings until the gland is so damaged that it can no longer fight back against the immune system attacking it with auto-antibodies.

QUESTION TWENTY-NINE

Can Thyroid Hormone Therapy cause Adjustment Side Effects?

This article is derived from a forum post I made in 2005. ---

It's good to see you on here on the forum again but I am sorry it is because you are not feeling well (per your post). I too had worsening of hypothyroid symptoms after starting thyroid hormone replacement medication.

I was so disappointed because I knew just the opposite was supposed to happen. On many of the websites I've researched, they talk about the introduction of medication with many patients, actually causing the thyroid to atrophy (cut back it's own production of hormone), so that even though you are putting hormone into the body from the outside, for a while you only break even, or even lose ground with your levels.

Sometimes it takes more than just the few weeks that they blood-retest a patient, for this altered level-change to show up. The TSH is suppressed immediately because there are more thyroid hormones (T4 and T3) in the blood stream but by the time the body actually utilizes that extra hormone, the levels start dropping again and a dosage increase is needed all over again! Others on this forum, have experienced this as I have and some are even just now getting increased on their dosages. It is very frustrating because the process seems to take so long! Your breathing trouble could be pressure on the trachea from swelling of your thyroid, according to what I have also read or could just be hypo-lack of thyroid hormone (oxygen hunger), slowing down your vital signs.

I do know that the constipation alone CAN MAKE YOU FEEL SICK. In fact you need to keep trying to find a solution to it because it can become toxic at some point if it becomes very severe. This happened to a nephew of mine and he became very ill due to it. Your symptoms, including the constipation, certainly do sound like hypothyroidism. Given time however and proper dose adjustments, you should see better days ahead, soon.

QUESTION THIRTY

Can Chemical Sensitivities happen with Autoimmune Thyroiditis?

The brief article following was a forum reply I made to a thyroid disease patient who found that they had negative after-effects from consuming alcohol. ---

Thyroid disease does cause increased chemical sensitivities in some patients, in fact they call it "Multiple Chemical Sensitivities" (MCS). I know since having Hashimoto's, I have extreme sensitivities to caffeine and chocolate.

Eighty-Seven Thyroid Disease Questions Answered!

I always had some sensitivity to these but it worsened with thyroid disease. It could be that you had a more severe reaction to alcohol (per your post) because of your thyroid disease. I also have sensitivity to alcohol, which I discovered kind of inadvertently. I drink very occasionally (infrequently) and in June-2005, my wife and I celebrated our 22nd anniversary with a bottle of Champagne (rare for us). I admit I finished-off the bottle because it was not a large size and had low alcohol content for a wine product and I started feeling sick afterward, which lasted several days! In my old days, before I reformed (LOL), I could drink most people under the table. I'll never do those things again, since becoming a Christian, plus I have no desire to become intoxicated on chemicals of any kind but I know for certain that the reaction I had was a result of the thyroid disease, among other possible factors involving health disorders I have co morbid to my Hashimoto's thyroiditis(i.e. Metabolic syndrome, pre-diabetic conditions) . Conditions such as adrenal fatigue, Mitral Valve Prolapse (heart murmur), fatty liver disease and Chronic Fatigue Syndrome can cause MCS as a feature of them as well.

SECTION THREE:
Questions and Answers THIRTY-ONE through FOURTY-FIVE

QUESTION THIRTY-ONE

Any Personal Experience with Adrenal Fatigue Co-morbid to Thyroid Disease?

When I was diagnosed with hypothyroidism, my readings according to the doctor were only "sub-clinical", with a TSH of "8.3" (range 0.4 to 4.8) and a T-3 Uptake flagged low. The rest of my thyroid hormone levels were in the lower half of normal. It wasn't until two years later I got the thyroid antibodies ones tested and my TG ABs were "537" (normal being <40) and my TPO ABs were "120" (normal being <35), so this was the test that actually confirmed Hashimoto's thyroiditis (autoimmune hypothyroidism).

My problem from the beginning, after I started my thyroid hormone replacement medication, was the fact that some of my symptoms actually WORSENED.

I was frustrated, so did an inline search using "Worse symptoms after starting thyroid replacement medication" as my search term (or something to that effect). It took me to sites stating that if you have UNTREATED adrenal insufficiency, this can worsen if you start thyroid hormone medication. This was also stated on the thyroid brand maker's websites! I decided I would get checked for "cortisol" levels -- it being the major "stress hormone" that regulates glucose and stress-levels in the body, among other things! I searched and found "Great Smokies Diagnostic Laboratories", who put out BodyBalance-StressChek Brand, home saliva tests at the time, to check DHEA/Cortisol levels. These are as accurate as blood tests, according to medical research groups. My DHEA was about mid-range but my cortisol on 4-different tests I took over a year period, were all either low-normal, borderline low and one was clinically low. I then found another company that sets up blood testing for LabOne and I had a 24-hour urine cortisol test done. The range on the urine test was <119 for males age-18 and older and my result was "10.7"! I finally made it to an actual Dr. visit and showed him these readings. As I suspected, he patronized me a bit but went ahead and sent me for an "ACTH Stimulation Test" (Expensive for a self-pay patient but highly diagnostic).

I was VERY ANXIOUS when I had the test done, which probably gave a falsely high "baseline cortisol level". They first get your baseline or starting level, and then inject you with ACTH - the hormone, that stimulates your adrenals to produce cortisol. They then rechecked my cortisol at 30-minute and 1-hour intervals. My baseline was "10.7", my 30-min reading was "25.7" and my 1-hour reading was "37.4". So, I passed the stimulation of my adrenals quite well BUT this DID NOT change the fact that my cortisol levels were low, without stimulation!

There is some reason for my low adrenal output of cortisol and I suspect it to be "adrenal fatigue", triggered by autoimmune thyroid disease. My symptoms have been; orthostatic hypotension (temporary dizziness/pressure in head when first standing) slow resting heartbeat, low resting blood pressure, fatigue, joint pain, post exertion fatigue (after physical activity), all of which I originally attributed to my thyroid disease. I do know that some of this worsened with my thyroid hormone medication treatment but I still need it or I risk worse hypothyroid symptoms that can result in severe consequences if left untreated.

Eighty-Seven Thyroid Disease Questions Answered!

I have instead added adrenal support supplements when I need them, to help with times of symptom flares from adrenal fatigue that occur due to fluctuations of low adrenal cortisol levels.

QUESTION THIRTY-TWO

Are there Similarities between Overactive Adrenals and a Hyperactive Thyroid?

My reply to a forum post regarding: "Overactive Adrenals Versus Hyperactive Thyroid".---

ACTH (Adrenocortitrophic hormone) is the hormone the pituitary gland releases to stimulate the adrenal gland to release more cortisol, just like TSH is released by the pituitary gland, to stimulate the thyroid to release more T-4 and T-3. The problem is, that too-much ACTH also means overproduction of cortisol That means your adrenal glands are overactive (Cushings Syndrome) when this is happening. That is why your blood and/or urine cortisol reading will be above the normal range.

Eighty-Seven Thyroid Disease Questions Answered!

Your Dr. will try to determine if it is caused possibly by a tumor in the pituitary gland or other cause. Don't let this scare you because just like a thyroid tumor (hot nodule) can cause the thyroid gland to overproduce (Graves' Disease), a pituitary or even adrenal tumor can also cause overproduction of the hormones they stimulate production-of (cortisol, ACTH, DHEA etc...). If there is a tumor, it is very rare that it would be cancerous, just like it is rare for thyroid tumors/nodules to be cancerous. They usually control these imbalances with medication but of course only a qualified Dr. can determine this through further diagnostic testing.

So, in a nutshell, they want to reduce your elevated cortisol if it becomes elevated for the preceding described reasons or from other causes, which results in "Cushings Disease" symptoms (excessive cortisol levels). Do an online search to learn more about this by going to a search-engine and placing the term "Symptoms of Cushings Disease", in the search bar. I personally had the "ACTH Stimulation test" administered (a measure of adrenal function, when stimulated) and not just my "ACTH" levels measured (pituitary hormone that stimulates adrenal output of cortisol).

My adrenals do under-produce adequate cortisol but not severe enough to be called "Addison's Disease" (opposite of Cushings), meaning too little cortisol, which does cause me symptoms of adrenal fatigue/exhaustion at times. I believe the medications they use to treat Cushing's patients are what they call cortisol-inhibitors but they do also try to remove any tumor they might find in the pituitary gland that may be causing the hormone imbalance.

As far as thyroid tumors/nodules go, I think the reason most of the time, they don't remove them (unless suspected of malignancy) is because thyroid hormone is easier to replace if hindered by a nodule. This, as opposed to trying to replace all of the hormones the pituitary is responsible for sending out to the other endocrine glands (hormone producing) in the body. Also, the kind of tumors that cause excessive hormone production are more dangerous than ones that cause inhibited hormone production such as in hypothyroidism. Tumors that Graves' Disease people have (overactive thyroid glands) do result in more surgeries to remove them than do the kind that are found in patients with Hashimoto's thyroiditis (under active thyroid glands).

They also sometimes "ablate" (destroy) the thyroid glands of Grave's patients because hyperthyroidism is more immediately dangerous, due to its effects in causing increased heart rate and blood pressure.

This is kind of the same problem with the Cushings disease scenario, which is 'sometimes' more immediately risky than Addison's because it causes excessive hormone levels in the body. With Addison's -- adrenal gland inadequacy, it is kind of like hypothyroidism. All they are required to do, is replace the low hormones, as determined by blood testing all levels that might be affected but with Cushing's (adrenal), as in Grave's (thyroid), they need to remove the cause of the over-production, so that damage does not occur to other organs in the body.

QUESTION THIRTY-THREE

Can Thyroid Disease Affect Speech?

From my forum reply regarding: "Can Thyroid Disease Affect Speech?".---

I'm willing to bet that sometimes people looking into this forum and others for thyroid disease support - maybe even Dr.s, who happen-by to read the postings, think that we are attributing too many things to thyroid disease but - here goes again! Some medical websites actually mention "difficulty pronouncing words", as a possible symptom of thyroid disease. There is a woman who has an interesting website, her name is "Sonja Midtlien", she is Norwegian and if you will put her name into the search-bar of www.google.com, I'm sure her thyroid website will be listed, for you to click on and go to, for browsing/reading.

She mentions that the "Norwegian Thyroid Association", lists "difficulty pronouncing words", as a symptom of Hashimoto's-Hypothyroidism and they state that the cause is "due to enlargement of the root of the tongue". That's their words, not mine, so everyone out there can take it for what it's worth!

Eighty-Seven Thyroid Disease Questions Answered!

We do know our thyroid gland regulates EVERYTHING in our body (metabolism), so it would not be hard to believe that speech can be affected in my opinion.

QUESTION THIRTY-FOUR

Is Asking your Doctor for Thyroid antibodies Testing Okay?

From my forum reply Re: "Asking your Doctor for Thyroid antibodies Testing".---

If you find your initial blood results at home (if you asked for copies) and you don't see that they tested you for thyroid antibodies levels, I would ask them to add this to your future ordered tests when you can. I'm not telling you what to do, it's just a suggestion because many Doctors for some reason don't test hypothyroid patients for thyroid antibodies (The "Anti-Thyroglobulin and Anti-Thyroperoxidase") and these are the ones that tell you if it is autoimmune hypothyroidism or not.

People with Hashimoto's thyroiditis (most common autoimmune cause in industrialized countries) have to monitor for any new sets of symptoms, worsening ones etc... because they are at increased risk for other autoimmune diseases, such as rheumatoid arthritis, adrenal insufficiency, diabetes, etc..., so if a Dr. says "it doesn't make any difference what kind of hypothyroidism you have or what is causing it", I would tend to disagree with him. In my opinion IT DOES MATTER what is causing a thyroid hormone imbalance and it's your body - you have a RIGHT to know what types of disease-processes are going on in it. The doctor-patient relationship should be reasonably open, so that patients don't feel intimidated if their Dr. seems reluctant to work with them, in establishing a cause for their under active thyroid gland. He may be the type that does listen, although I don't mean to pre-judge (there are certainly many great Dr.s out there), I just wanted to prepare you for what most of us out here have been through, in having to suggest or even sometimes "demand" that testing be ordered to further evaluate our thyroid disease cases. We refer to this as being a "proactive patient" and studies have shown that activated patients are the ones who have better treatment outcomes.

QUESTION THIRTY-FIVE

Can Hashimoto's Thyroiditis cause Anxiety and Depression?

From my forum reply regarding the question - "Can Hashimoto's Thyroiditis cause Anxiety and Depression?". ---

Yes, you can have both anxiety and depressive symptoms with hypothyroidism, especially if it is the autoimmune type (Hashimoto's Thyroiditis). Most of us on this forum can relate to this because we have experienced this. Sometimes I'm concerned that it always sounds like I'm knocking Dr.s and I really don't mean to come across that way but some Dr.s believe that just because your lab ranges are normal on blood retests you have done, to monitor your thyroid hormone therapy, that this means you should also feel "normal". The fact is however, that progressive hypothyroidism that has an autoimmune cause (i.e. Hashimoto's thyroiditis) can make you swing back and forth between hypothyroid and hyperthyroid symptoms, including aspects of low mood and anxiety and sometimes these episodes may become mixed.

Eighty-Seven Thyroid Disease Questions Answered!

I had a severe anxiety phase just before I became progressively hypothyroid with my own Hashimoto's thyroiditis. A little better explanation is this: When the thyroid is being damaged by "antibodies", it will cause it to release spurts of too much hormone, as a defense mechanism but as soon as this overdrive mode stops, you drop back down to low levels again and after a while, the thyroid becomes so damaged, it cannot recover or fight off the autoimmune attack anymore and continues to slip down into progressive hypothyroidism.

I've heard a lot of people's stories about Hashimoto's Disease/hypothyroidism and they related having anxiety attacks when they had too many duties to perform and it overwhelmed them (stress-induced) and other times it just happened to them for no apparent reason (possibly hormone fluctuations). Have you had the "thyroid antibodies" tests (i.e. the TPO and TG antibodies)? You might consider this because it can reveal an autoimmune attack going on, even when thyroid hormone levels are in normal-range.

QUESTION THIRTY-SIX

Any Comments on Thyroid Hormone Therapy and Depression Symptoms?

From my forum reply Re: "Thyroid Hormone Therapy and Depression Symptoms".---

By going to www.thyroid.about.com – website, you then can put in search words such as "Depression and Thyroid Disease" in the search-bar that appears at top-page and it will list articles you can click on. I do know there is a belief by some medical experts that depressive thyroid patients need t-3 hormone and not the t-4 only, which is what Synthroid, among other brands contain (needing t-3 may not be the case with everyone who has depression). Most, if not all of us who are hypothyroid patients have had depression with our thyroid disorders. Mine completely lifted when my hormone therapy was increased to the correct dose (my TSH needs suppressed to under 1.0) but that's me and who's to say that's right for each person who suffers stubborn depression symptoms. It's worth researching though and I hope the website I suggested helps you with information in regard to this issue.

Eighty-Seven Thyroid Disease Questions Answered!

Please also communicate with someone, including posting on thyroid support forums, when you feel down.

In former posts, I speak of my problem with the "antidepressant prescribing craze" but I hope no one thinks I am advocating against SSRI antidepressants themselves. My mother takes Prozac, plus is treated for her underactive thyroid and she does very well. My problem is use of these drugs to treat unrelieved emotional symptoms when thyroid treatment is not optimized, especially when this alone could be the answer for some people (getting optimal thyroid dose levels). If a patient is not optimized and they are placed on an antidepressant, I am concerned about their being able to distinguish the side-effects of the antidepressant, from any unrelieved thyroid symptoms. I hope that makes sense. However, some people need help on an immediate basis and if they know their thyroid hormone medication is at the correct level, an antidepressant might be exactly what they need! No two situations are exactly the same but GENERALLY, making sure thyroid dose is optimal, is usually a good idea before accepting a prescribed mood disorder drug that is usually a long-term or lifelong treatment.

QUESTION THIRTY-SEVEN

What are Natural and Synthetic T4 and T3 Hormone Therapies?

From my forum reply Re: "Natural and Synthetic T4 and T3 Hormone Therapies" ---

Levothyroxine is one name for synthetic t-4 hormone replacement medication, which comes in the different brands such as "Synthroid, Levoxyl, Levothroid" etc... They are basically the same thing but some of these are considered generics and many doctors prefer to stick to the major brands, due to generics sometimes being 'less potent' at same dose-levels. I started out on Synthroid but I didn't get the expected relief of symptoms, so my Doctor placed me on a combo t-3/t-4 hormone called "Armour Thyroid", which is a natural version, made from animal thyroid glands – porcine/pigs. Natural brands of thyroid hormone are used for the same thing that these other synthetic types are used for which is -- thyroid hormone replacement for hypothyroid patients.

Eighty-Seven Thyroid Disease Questions Answered!

The Doctor who first treated me for hypothyroidism, switched me from the synthetic T-4 only brand I had been taking for about a year, thinking I might have a problem with t-4 to t-3 conversion (a process that occurs naturally in the body but fails to do so in some patients). He switched me, believing I might be a person with inability in my body, to convert t-4 only hormone into the other needed t-3 (more active) hormone. This suspicion was due to my experiencing unrelieved symptoms, while being on the brand hormone I was started on (Synthroid). Most people don't have a problem with this and looking back I have a feeling mine was more of an "insufficient dose" problem rather than an "impaired conversion" one, because my blood TSH level (test used to monitor the therapy) was not suppressed adequately by my dose. Reputable medical sources state that TSH is supposed to be brought down to between 1.0 and 2.0 for proper treatment of hypothyroid patients (TSH elevates with hypothyroidism) and mine was only suppressed down to between 3.0 and 5.0 for at least that first year I was treated.

QUESTION THIRTY-EIGHT

Do you have more Information on Emotional Symptoms and Hypothyroid Treatment?

This article is a forum-response I made Re: "Emotional Symptoms and Hypothyroid Treatment"---

Most of us can relate to most of your symptoms and to the depression which is very common with hypothyroidism. I'm an age-42 man (as of year 2006), who went from going to the Dr. maybe once every 5 or 6 years, to going very frequently due to sudden worsening of symptoms that actually started years earlier. It was extremely depressing and caused me great anxiety as well, to go from a strong (6ft 215lb), hard working man, to feeling like I could barely walk across a room. I admit now that I actually did become suicidal at times. By being patient in getting dosage adjustments in treating my hypothyroidism and especially with God's help, I made it through those incredibly tough times. I still have symptom flares and generally have more fatigue at times than I used-to but I have improved in many other areas!

Please always talk to someone -- and us too at the forum when you need to (corresponding with fellow patients who go through the same things you do). Just put "need help now!" or something to that effect and we'll correspond with you as quickly as we can. Let me also encourage you by saying that you will see improvement over time, with thyroid hormone therapy, to treat your hypothyroidism though it seems hard to see right now! You have a doctor who is trying you on increased doses and he will keep doing so until you feel better and are in the right range for you to feel better on your hormone replacement level! It is so hard to be patient but once you start gaining ground, you will see happiness slowly return and in turn it will bring back your ambition!

Myself and others I've read posts from on this forum, have had the same experience with symptoms being claimed by their doctors, not to be thyroid-related (especially emotional ones), when we know for a fact they are. Yes, it is very frustrating. It is also insulting for lingering symptoms to be called psychosomatic (imagined). Many times I actually believe it is simply a matter of what's easier for some doctors to treat and that's why the emotional diagnosis is used a lot.

Of course there are those who would disagree with this and they have that right -- but I've read so many testimonies of people who went through this and once they had proper treatment for their thyroid disease, the symptoms finally resolved. It usually amounted to finding the right doctor or in the patient finally influencing the doctor toward better treatment options (i.e. dose increases or changing brands).

QUESTION THIRTY-NINE

Is there Risk for Crohn's Disease in thyroid Patients?

This short reply, I made, was to a thyroid patient who was having stomach symptoms, including blood in their stools and symptoms affecting their eyes – Re: "The Risk for Crohn's Disease in thyroid Patients" ---

I've not seen these symptoms mentioned for hypothyroidism before and they do sound serious, needing a doctor's care and investigation.

Eighty-Seven Thyroid Disease Questions Answered!

Most of us have the autoimmune type of hypothyroidism, called Hashimoto's Thyroiditis and as I have researched, found that one autoimmune disease can lead to another, so they can co-exist but this would be the only connection I would see, generally.

There is a colon disease called "Crohn's" and I know a man who has this and it too is an autoimmune disease. He had bleeding as you described and it also caused him anemia but with treatment, his is in remission and has been for several years now.

Of course I don't know if you have this or even a similar condition but this is an example of a type disease that can cause this and that thyroid patients are at slightly increased risk for developing. This friend I referred to, also did mention to me that the Crohn's seriously affected his eyes and is also why I mentioned it as a possibility in your case, that your doctor may want to investigate. I hope you find a good physician that can get to the definitive cause and administer the treatment you need soon!

QUESTION FORTY

Can Thyroid Cysts and Hypothyroid Symptoms mean Hashimoto's?

From my forum-reply re: "Thyroid Cysts and Hypothyroid Symptoms can mean Hashimoto's" ---

(My reply was to a forum-poster who described having hypothyroid symptoms and a soft lump on their thyroid gland that could be felt on the outside of their throat.)

The symptoms you described can be thyroid related and related directly to your cyst as well. The cyst may actually be what they call a "cystic nodule". Nodules happen in both Hashimoto's Thyroiditis (Hypothyroidism-under active) and in Graves Disease (Hyperthyroidism-overactive). However, since you have spells of both hyperthyroid type symptoms and hypothyroid type symptoms, it could be the Hashimoto's type of thyroid autoimmunity because with Hashimoto's a person can go through periods of switching back and forth between both types of symptoms for a while, usually early into the disease, before becoming permanently hypothyroid.

Eighty-Seven Thyroid Disease Questions Answered!

It is the thyroid's way of trying to fight off the autoimmune attack, by temporarily increasing its hormone output in attempt to overwhelm the damage and inflammation occurring from antibodies, mistakenly sent from the immune system to attack it.

I would get the "antibodies" blood tests done that can detect autoimmune thyroid disease along with thyroid hormone levels (thyroid panel) because Hashimoto's can exist in people even when hormones are within normal range. Don't let a Dr. tell you otherwise because it is an established fact, confirmed by reputable medical sources. Unfortunately some Dr.s actually don't know this (an unfortunate fact). The antibody tests are the "Anti-Thyroglobulin (TG) and Anti-thyroidperoxidase (TPO)" Tests. I would tell the doctor that you want these done and be firm in requesting the tests, not letting him talk you out of them being done. Let us know the results that come back on your tests if you like and we'll add follow up comments if your antibodies do happen to be elevated.

QUESTION FOURTY-ONE

Any Suggestions Regarding the Thyroid Patient – Doctor Dilemma?

This article is derived from my post Re: "The Thyroid Patient – Doctor Dilemma".---

Many other thyroid patients, posting on forums have attested to experiencing some of the same disappointing things with certain Dr.s they have been-to, as I have. If it were just a few people reporting these type things in regard to botched thyroid disease treatments, you might say it wasn't a serious problem but I've heard it constantly from a lot of people for many years now. All five Dr.s I first visited for treatment of my thyroid disease, wanted to prescribe me antidepressants (two gave out samples) and except for that first Dr. who prescribed them (I tried them for about 2-months), I threw them all away if prescribed afterward, starting with samples. My problem-symptoms were joint pain and fatigue but I expressed plainly that if I did have anxiety/depression, it was very mild and a result, rather than a cause of my symptoms.

This was all after I started thyroid hormone replacement medication and had gotten well-past the emotional symptoms. I had only the lingering physical symptoms to deal with at that point, which was due to insufficient hormone dose levels.

After the first two Dr.s prescribed these psychotropic drugs on several visits to each of them, as I sought help for my fibromyalgia type pain, my wife asked to go with me just to see if the next doctor I changed to, in attempt to get better help, would do this as well. She was flabbergasted when he also tried to push these drugs on me within the first 30 secs of that first office visit. When I changed to a yet another new doctor again later, she was with me again at the office visit, when he too immediately reached for the script-pad to prescribe an SSRI antidepressant. My family, my parents, my friends etc... all knew I did not have emotional issues and in fact I was very optimistic and improved greatly in that area. The drugs were offered simply because I had unrelieved physical symptoms and this apparently was not what these doctors wanted to hear and was an obvious frustration to them. My TSH level the first time I complained of no relief from my thyroid hormone therapy was "4.98" Reference range was 0.5 to 5.0 .

After I complained that my dose was too low via search I did on proper TSH levels, my doctor increased my dose to suppress my TSH down to "3.10". This was over nearly two years period of time but each time they would say "YOU'RE IN THE NORMAL RANGE", there's no reason you shouldn't be completely well. In the mean time, I had all those tests I listed in earlier posts and for all of that time, I SIMPLY NEEDED A DOSE INCREASE and my symptoms would have improved. The most reputable medical sources in existence, including the U.S. National Institutes of Health recommend that TSH levels be suppressed down to between "1.0 and 3.0", in treating hypothyroidism with thyroid hormone dosing.

What I discovered was that these less-informed doctors actually believed that ANYTHING within the normal values range (for diagnosing rather than treating hypothyroidism) was acceptable. They called my remaining symptoms psychosomatic because they did not know about the importance of optimizing treatment (dose-titration) and it was easier for them to prescribe an SSRI antidepressant, rather than adjusting my dose to accomplish this optimization.

Eighty-Seven Thyroid Disease Questions Answered!

I spent a ton of unnecessary money for tests to diagnose other possible causes of my symptoms, when adequate dosing was what I was lacking and in need of.

Some people suggest that this type of scenario that is happening to patients is due to over-booking of office visits and high medical liability insurance costs for doctors. I'm sure these are two of the major reasons but it is still a terrible thing to be experienced by patients regardless of these factors. It is people like us who are free to express our grievances that can make a difference for others in the future, who are suffering these type things and I hope reform of these problems will someday take place. It won't happen any time soon if the problem is not recognized by those who have the authority to help it change for the better.

QUESTION FOURTY-TWO

Is there a way to distinguish between Good Thyroid Doctors versus Bad Ones?

From my post Re: "Good Thyroid Doctors Versus Bad Ones". ---

My Mother has a Dr. that is absolutely sensational! He is not cold and indifferent but actually listens to patients without patronizing them. I have tried to get in with him several times, over several years but he is booked-up and there is a long waiting list. Other experiences I've had with past Dr.s were pathetic and I don't know any other way to express a bad experience other than to tell it "the way it was". To not warn people about the "obvious things" that are happening, such as people being treated with antidepressants, when the root cause is untreated or under-treated thyroid disease or because of other serious, undiagnosed health disorders, would be as a disservice to them. It would also be a disservice to not give them good information in regard to qualified thyroid doctors who are out there (Mary Shomon does this on her personal thyroid information website).

If we suggest something to possibly research and look into as fellow-patients through forums, it might be more of a process of elimination, than the actual answer but it can still be helpful on many different levels. The people posting on patient support forums KNOW we are fellow patients and we try to give as many views as we can without getting too outrageous (our knowledge is limited but some things are obvious). In my opinion, I would rather have several possibilities to research-out than only one "iffy one" suggested by a doctor who has not taken time to thoroughly evaluate my case. I had Doctors suggest possibilities for unrelieved symptoms in my case, including Rheumatoid Arthritis (ruled-out by an "RA Factor test"), Gout (ruled-out by "Uric Acid Test"), Low-Testosterone (ruled by blood and saliva testing), Diabetes (ruled-out by "glucose-average 90 day test – A1C"), Addison's Disease (ruled-out by "ACTH Stimulation Test"), Allergies (ruled-out by "blood-allergens tests"), etc.... This was AFTER being on thyroid medication for over two years but through research on my own, I found that I was not in the optimal TSH range to feel better from my thyroid hormone therapy, so I increased my dose through a new doctor and "Presto!" I got much better (monitored closely with blood retests)!

Eighty-Seven Thyroid Disease Questions Answered!

It was other thyroid patients who warned me about the possibility of "under-treatment" and that it was a fairly common problem but 2-Doctors actually laughed at me when I suggested under-treatment and they basically said "leave the treatment to us". How wonderful it would have been if I could have actually done that and been properly diagnosed and treated earlier and saved all that money, as a self-pay, uninsured patient! HINDSIGHT is an advantage and is exactly what patients who've been through this type thing have on their side, that they can warn others patients about! To not share the pitfalls along with the positives is like giving only half an answer to a question of great importance. Thank God for the excellent Dr.s who are out there! They are to be praised! But, patients desperately need to recognize inferior treatment when it does happen, so that they can exercise their right to a second opinion.

QUESTION FOURTY-THREE

Is Thyroid Patient Education and Proactiveness Important?

This article is derived from my post Re: "Thyroid Patient Education and Proactiveness".---

I just recently found information about hot and cold nodules (thyroid tumors) and the "hot" ones can cause the thyroid to continually release hormone and causes hyperthyroidism similar to what Graves' disease people have (autoimmune hyperthyroidism – overactive). A nodule, may cause transient hyperthyroidism for a while, like Hashimoto's thyroiditis people have (autoimmune hypothyroidism – under active, preceded by temporary hyperthyroidism) when the thyroid is fizzling out but then becomes a "cold nodule" and no longer elevates hormone production from the gland. Since you've had hypothyroid readings and high antibodies (per your post), yours is almost certainly the Hashimoto's kind of thyroid autoimmunity and is also why the doctor didn't see a need in further scanning your gland (radioactive imaging) at this point.

There is a site created by a Hashimoto's-Man called "hateshopping" (not certain if the site is still up or if it is under a new domain-name now) and if you are able to go there, click on his article titled "WHY YOU ARE NOT CRAZY". He has other very good ones too but in this one he relates how Dr.s misdiagnosed him as "Bi-Polar, Schizophrenic" etc..., in other words, the old "psychosomatic" catch-all diagnoses, rather than blood testing him for possible diseases, including thyroid – the one he was eventually diagnosed with. He also relates on the site, having had hyperthyroid symptoms with his Hashimoto's, with rapid heart beat and elevated blood pressure. He too knocks negative experiences he's had with Dr.s but he also mentions there are many out there who are trustworthy.

YES, I admit I've been very passionate in trying to inform others about the importance of patient proactive-ness and self-education because of mine, my wife's, my mother's, my uncle's etc.... - experiences in not getting diagnosed properly, without the tremendous added expense of changing Dr.s, wrong tests being ordered, etc.... This is why I SO APPRECIATE thyroid patient advocates like Mary Shomon.

Eighty-Seven Thyroid Disease Questions Answered!

She has a book called "Living Well With Hypothyroidism", and I highly recommend it and her other book "Living Well With Autoimmune Disease". NO, she's not a Doctor but the following are examples of Dr.s who endorsed her books: Stephen Langer MD, Marie Savard MD, Larian Gillespie MD, Carol Roberts MD, David Brownstien MD,etc... What do you know – a thyroid patient with experience and knowledge!

Also: Dr. Lowe is Director of Research for the "Fibromyalgia Research Foundation" and has a "B.A., M.A., B.S., and a doctorate in Chiropractic medicine. His education far exceeds that needed to be a Chiropractic Dr. and thankfully research like the foundation he is involved in, is ongoing for fibromyalgia and thyroid patients. His research agrees with that by many other Dr.s and researchers like "Mary Shomon", who is not a Dr. but is recognized by the medical community as one of the leading authorities on thyroid disease. She has a series of books on the subject, endorsed by many Dr.s as previously mentioned. I personally, will take good information from any source I can get and I always confirm it by my own research of other reputable sources that compare with it.

QUESTION FOURTY-FOUR

Is Diagnosing and Monitoring Thyroid Disease by Blood the Best Way?

From my post Re: "Diagnosing and Monitoring Thyroid Disease by Blood".---

Doctors after all these years of advancement in thyroid disease diagnosis and treatments, should know that people with autoimmune thyroid diseases (Both Hashimoto's thyroiditis and Graves' disease), can have full blown symptoms even when hormone lab-ranges are still within normal range. Many reputable medical sites state that "high antibody levels" prevent thyroid hormones from binding to receptor sites (process of taking them into the cells of the body to regulate metabolism), even when hormone levels are adequate, causing hypothyroidism symptoms. They especially should know that the TSH test alone will miss a lot of borderline cases of developing thyroid disease as well – especially those that are developing due to antibodies attacking the thyroid gland (autoimmunity).

That would be right at almost 4-weeks (per your post) for a new thyroid hormone dose to take effect and this is supposed to be long enough for it to change your lab ranges as much as it's going to but some doctors allow for 6 to 8 weeks to make certain. When I go for retesting of my thyroid hormone levels, to monitor my therapy, I will usually only skip the dose for that morning until the blood is drawn, then take it afterward because thyroid hormone has at least a few hours half life (the natural type/brands like Armour) and the synthetic (like Synthroid) has a half life of several days, so should still be built up in your system and not cause much problem by delaying a dose on one day. It is my opinion however, and Dr.s may actually disagree with this, that taking a thyroid hormone dose the same morning, just before blood is drawn for a retest, may show inaccurately/falsely high medication levels because it hasn't been absorbed into the cells of the body yet and is still mostly in the blood stream. The makers of Armour actually suggest on their website, delaying your dose on the morning of a blood draw.

QUESTION FOURTY-FIVE

What are the Far-Reaching Effects of Thyroid Antibodies?

This article is from my forum post Re: "The Far-Reaching Effects of Thyroid Antibodies".---

I've researched about "Sub-Acute Thyroiditis" but understood it to be temporary as you stated and I don't believe it causes the elevated antibodies you have, as stated on your post. I could be wrong about that, so you might try a search on it using that name of your illness but I'm fairly certain it doesn't typically cause thyroid antibodies to develop or at least not to significant (flagged high) levels.

I have Hashimoto's Hypothyroidism but I didn't have an antibodies test for two years, I only knew my thyroid was low functioning. I finally had an antibodies tests, May of this year (2005) and my TOP ABs were "120" (normal being <35) and my TG ABs were "537" (normal being <40). My Doctor indicated that high antibody levels can cause symptoms even when thyroid hormone levels are at normal-range and I researched this fact and found lots of confirming information on it.

Eighty-Seven Thyroid Disease Questions Answered!

I also found studies in which many Dr.s believe fibromyalgia and Chronic Fatigue Syndrome are often thyroid-related. I hope yours is the temporary type of thyroiditis but with those antibody levels, it looks like Hashimoto's thyroiditis – the permanent type that eventually results in progressive hypothyroidism.

Thyroid patient Advocate - Mary Shomon is a Hashimoto's sufferer and recognized as one of the nations top authorities on the subject. She did a survey (Quality of Life Survey of Thyroid Patients) in 2003 and results have just recently been released. A group of 860 Hypo/Hashi people, with TSH levels in optimal range, reported still having symptoms as follows: 789 (92%) still had fatigue/exhaustion despite treatment. Over 500 still had weight gain/unable to lose. 437 still had joint/muscle pain etc.... It is a very revealing survey in regard to this disease and the effectiveness of treatment for it (sill we need it or would suffer even more severe consequences). My belief is that antibody levels cause the lingering symptoms in some patients, so we need diet exercise and all-around better practices in taking care of ourselves to help improve them, in addition to our thyroid hormone replacement therapy.

SECTION FOUR:
Questions and Answers FOURTY-SIX through SIXTY

QUESTION FOURTY-SIX

Any Ideas Regarding Highly Elevated Thyroid Antibodies and Steroid Treatment?

From my forum post regarding "Highly Elevated Thyroid Antibodies and Steroid Treatment".---

The ATHYP abbreviation you asked about, means Anti-Thyro-Peroxidase Antibodies test (also sometimes abbreviated simply "TPO") and the ATHYG means Anti-Thyro-Globulin Antibodies test (also sometimes abbreviated simply "TG"). If your TPO ABs were elevated but not the TG ones, this still means autoimmune thyroid disease most likely because some people only have one or the other elevated and some have both elevated.

The corticosteroid treatment you mention is sometimes given short-term to reduce inflammation in patients who appear to have a high level of it.

Eighty-Seven Thyroid Disease Questions Answered!

It is a hydrocortisone steroid, like "Prednisone", which a Dr. gave me short-term, in my own case, when he saw I had high antibody readings of both types, that he thought might be contributing to my joint pain. These corticosteroids are given for many inflammatory diseases, sometimes short term and sometimes long term (such as for rheumatoid arthritis, Addison's Disease etc...) As was my case, doctors may give steroid treatment to patients, if they feel they are at risk for Hashimoto's Encephalitis (HE), which is a severe and sometimes life-threatening neurological response to elevated thyroid antibodies.

My TPO Antibodies were "120" (range at the lab was <35) and my TG Antibodies were "537" (Range at the lab was <45), so in my case, the anti-thyroglobulin ABs were much higher than the anti-peroxidase ones, although they were considerably above normal too. It's strange that labs vary on their normal ranges and sometimes, it's a matter of where they place the decimal point and whether they add one or not. Your test had a normal range on the TPO of <2, but I've seen ones that had "0-74" as the normal range (not sure why they vary from lab to lab). Yours would still be flagged "high" even at this higher normal range.

Hypothyroid patients even without HE, sometimes have neurological symptoms and I think Dr.s are now learning this to be more common than originally thought. There was a time I would wake up in the night, early into my own disease, feeling like I was having a little seizure and I would feel a strange pain on one side of my tongue, at the same time. It was a weird sensation but I felt sure it was the hypothyroidism, rather than hints of Hashimoto's Encephalitis because they also list "tingling and numbness in hands, arms, feet and legs" as a hypothyroid symptom on some medical sources. Encephalitis symptoms would be far worse than these.

QUESTION FOURTY-SEVEN

Any Suggestions for Dealing with Hashimoto's Disease and Hypothyroidism?

The following is derived from my forum post regarding "Dealing with Hashimoto's Disease and Hypothyroidism".---

I would say that your TSH of "8.87" is considerably elevated, but it is hard to give more specific feedback without knowing the ranges on the test. These are found on your results and look something like this - "Range: 0.4 to 4.0". I have read numerous articles that have listed soy (per your mention of soy in your diet) as a contributing factor to thyroid problems. Testing high for thyroid antibodies probably means you have Hashimotos Disease, which is a progressive autoimmune thyroiditis that over time will make your thyroid fail to function. You may have only noticed the fatigue symptom so far -- as you related, but you've probably had some symptoms you disregarded as being something like stress, aging or working to hard, just like the fatigue you mention as being "vague".

Hashimoto's disease can make your symptoms manifest as either hypothyroid (under active) or hyperthyroid (overactive) in its early stages but always becomes a progressive hypothyroid disease, eventually. Some of my own symptoms as a Hashimoto's – hypothyroid patient have been dry skin, heart flutters, fatigue, mind fog, forgetfulness, anxiety, etc... My best advice at this point is to stop the soy and start your prescribed hormone replacement medication. You may go through some strange feelings after starting the medication (adjustment symptoms) like heart flutters, maybe even some hair loss, but by continuing to take it, you will feel better over time. I also found information stating that soy can have negative affects on hypothyroid patients, being a "goitrogen food" (potentially lowers thyroid hormones and increases thyroid inflammation). Your antibodies are highly elevated, per your posted results. Your TSH @ 8.87 indicates your thyroid is already struggling to keep up with your body's hormone needs. Your T-4 is almost borderline-low, further proof your hormone levels are dropping from the autoimmune attack on your thyroid gland. Even your Thyroglobulin Antibodies (TG) are elevated but not near as much as the TPO – antithyroidperoxidase ones are.

It sounds like your Dr. has positively diagnosed you as having Hashimoto's disease. His advice to you sounds good about needing dose adjustments due to the antibodies being elevated because they will cause more damage to your thyroid over time. I've heard some sources on websites say that the antibodies also attack your replacement hormone as it enters your body but I'm not sure there is any medically-confirmed proof of that (this is mostly claimed about "natural" brands). Weight gain can definitely happen despite treatment and it is hard for me personally to lose weight, as a fellow thyroid patient. I'm 6ft., 215lb but can't seem to reduce from this and I will fluctuate up to 220 instead. I almost quit eating at one time out of frustration (not a good idea) and still didn't lose weight (Strange). I don't mind being big, since I'm a man but wanted more energy and any extra pounds does not help me in this area, so I continue to work on personal weight loss -- for the sake of overall health as well.

QUESTION FOURTY-EIGHT

Is Thyroid Autoimmunity – a Major Factor in Symptoms?

This article is from a post I made in regard to "Thyroid Autoimmunity – a Major Factor in Symptoms".---

I would like to say that I, like many thyroid patients, went through 5 Doctors before receiving a proper diagnosis. I was diagnosed with Generalized Anxiety Disorder, depression, psycho-somatic symptoms etc..., and It was due to my being given this run-around, that I finally insisted on diagnostic blood tests and the diagnosis of my thyroid disease (Hashimoto's-hypothyroidism) was properly made. What's funny is that I suggested "thyroid disorder" to that very first Dr. I visited with my symptoms because I knew beyond-doubt that my condition had a medical/physical cause, with emotional symptoms being only one aspect of it. There was a survey done by Thyroid Patient Advocate - Mary Shomon in 2003 of 1000 thyroid patients. I realize she is literally shunned by some in the Medical Community but is praised by just as many reputable people practicing in Medical field.

Eighty-Seven Thyroid Disease Questions Answered!

In this survey, which was the first and largest of its kind, over HALF of patients on thyroid replacement hormone therapy for hypothyroidism and with TSH ranges at optimal range, still had lingering symptoms such as joint pain, serious fatigue, depression etc... This tells me, it is neither the doctors nor the patients in many cases but is often the "autoimmune component" of thyroid disease itself that causes or contributes-to symptoms and not whether the thyroid hormones are treated to get them into the optimal range or not (this still should be done however). If symptoms that continue, even while on treatment, are so rare in treated thyroid patients, why would a survey of this sort and similar ones to it, have these type results. Why are SO MANY online patients with autoimmune thyroid disease, seemingly in the very same boat in regard to unsatisfactory symptom relief? Are there this many psycho-somatic people? No, but rather there are many patients who suffer from the effects of an autoimmune process that is affecting their body, causing inflammation and alterations in their immune system function. In my personal but firm opinion, this is the most important factor contributing to unsatisfactory results in some treated hypothyroid patients and there are medical research studies that point to this fact as well.

QUESTION FOURTY-NINE

Can Goiters occur with Hashimoto's Thyroiditis?

This article is derived from my forum post on the subject of "Goiters that can occur with Hashimoto's Thyroiditis". ---

Yes, it does sound like Hashimoto's disease (description of thyroid problem given by the forum-poster) although there is a type of "thyroiditis", called Painful Thyroiditis (subacute) -- a temporary condition that clears up after a while (4 to 6 weeks). I'm not saying yours will hurt permanently but a lot of Hashi's people have pain in their thyroid glands that comes and goes and varies in severity but never completely goes away. Other patients experience temporary pain in their glands once and after that, the pain never returns (usually true of subacute thyroiditis). Non-painful goiters and mildly painful goiters are fairly common with Hashimoto's thyroiditis. Some people have large swelling and never any pain, who knows for sure why it manifests differently among different patients. Other Hashi's patients never experience a significant goiter and some only develop small nodules and only mild goiters (me included).

Eighty-Seven Thyroid Disease Questions Answered!

If you've been diagnosed with hypothyroidism, it is almost certainly caused by lifetime thyroiditis (it's the most common cause in industrialized countries) and if you tested positive for antibodies, this helps confirm that the hypothyroidism is caused by autoimmune thyroiditis - Hashimoto's disease. You might do an online search on "Goiters Caused by Hashimoto's" and this will probably yield a lot of information. If you see cancerous nodules mentioned, don't let that scare you because it is rare (in less than 5% of cases) and if you know you have Hashi's, you know that's the cause of your nodules. I've had slight dull aches in my thyroid gland from time to time but no serious pain.

I may be sticking my neck out a little now but when I had a problem in the past getting a Dr. to order me antibodies tests with my having recurrent symptoms and dosage problems with my thyroid replacement medication, I found websites that set up blood testing/no with Dr. visit required. They send results directly to you and you simply have your blood drawn at one of their network of locations (usually doctor's offices that participate). There are several of these firms out there that offer the blood testing, which is completed by reputable labs, such as Quest or LabCorp.

The one I used was www.healthcheckusa.com (networking through LabCorp). The tests were also less expensive than I was able to get through my doctor's office or local hospital. They tell you the closest location you can have blood drawn at (within miles of you) and you get blood drawn there - no office visit required.

If you have a Dr. that refuses you a test, I would consider a firm like the one I describe above. There are many now out there, which helps people to have blood tests done that they find difficulty getting ordered through their doctors for whatever reasons.

QUESTION FIFTY

Any Comments on Adrenal Fatigue and Thyroid Hormone Therapy?

This is a forum post I made in 2005, regarding my experience with "Adrenal Fatigue and Thyroid Hormone Therapy".---

Back when I first was diagnosed with hypothyroidism, I didn't get the expected symptom relief from my thyroid hormone replacement therapy. Research I did on this problem and the potential causes of it, mentioned that LOW adrenal hormones (low cortisol) could worsen symptoms of adrenal insufficiency if you start thyroid hormone medication but do not first correct the hypo-cortisolism. As far as HIGH cortisol goes, there is probably an effect there as well because your thyroid and adrenal hormones interact and some medical sources even call it the "Thyroid-Adrenal-Axis". Clinically low cortisol is called "Addison's Disease" and high cortisol is called "Cushing's Disease" (use these terms to search these conditions online).

I did several home adrenal hormone saliva tests - four over a year period.

Eighty-Seven Thyroid Disease Questions Answered!

These showed I had consistently low cortisol levels but probably not severe enough to be called Addison's disease and more probably a sub-clinical but significant type of "Adrenal Fatigue" or adrenal exhaustion. None of my Dr.s took it seriously, so to this day I still have a degree of it that can come in flares and cause me concerning symptoms, including a lowered tolerance for stress (stressors). I had the 24-hour urine cortisol measure done as well, which also revealed that my level of the hormone was low. The range for adult males age 18 and over was <119 and my result was "10.7". Even my doctor at the time of the test, admitted my level was one of the lowest he had ever seen on a 24-hr urine cortisol test. Despite this fact, I am required to treat the adrenal fatigue myself with safe, natural adrenal-boosting supplements because doctors do not recognize low adrenal function unless it is severe enough to require cortisol replacement therapy (cortical steroid drugs).

QUESTION FIFTY-ONE

Is Getting Leveled-out on Thyroid Hormone Replacement Difficult?

Forum Post: "Getting Leveled-out on Thyroid Hormone Replacement".---

With your TSH going from 0.15 to 7.63, this definitely looks like Hashimoto's Disease (autoimmune hypothyroidism) because you are going from a hyperthyroid to a hypothyroid reading on blood labs, within a short space of time. If I understand correctly, Graves Disease causes a constant hyperthyroid state, so much so, that it endangers some people with severe cases, of having uncontrollable hypertension and tachycardia (rapid heart rate) and they end up having to remove or destroy their thyroid gland, followed by placing them on thyroid hormone therapy. Yours sure sounds like the often present 'swings' Hashimoto's patients have, early into the disease (from hyperthyroid to hypothyroid, called "Hashitoxicosis"). I too have had intermittent hyperthyroid times but mine declined into hypothyroidism fairly shortly after a few weeks of hyperthyroid symptoms and I then stayed hypothyroid from that time on.

Eighty-Seven Thyroid Disease Questions Answered!

I now take 150mg of Armour Thyroid brand hormone medication for my case.

Levoxyl is the name for synthetic T-4 (often prescribed via the Synthroid brand) and Dr.s usually prescribe it more often than the natural forms, the most well known natural type being Armour as I referred-to earlier, which is a combination of both T-3 & T-4. I was actually first started on Synthroid and switched to Armour by a doctor who thought the brand might be superior in my case. The problem in SOME PEOPLE is that their system won't naturally convert the T-4 only hormone, into enough of the other needed "T-3" hormone. They call this an "impaired hormone conversion problem". The T-3 is actually the more "active" form of thyroid hormone. Some people do just fine on the synthetic T-4 (my own mother does for example). On the other hand some people don't tolerate the natural Armour type medication because it causes them spells of hyperthyroid type symptoms (T3 sensitivity) but I've personally never had that problem. Another thing people aren't aware of (me included until I found out) is that when you take thyroid medication, your own thyroid cuts back on it's own production of hormone (atrophy of the gland).

This means if you are not taking a "full replacement dose", for a while you will just break-even and not experience immediate improvement in low thyroid symptoms. That's why Dr.s have you re-test several times especially at the beginning of administering a new dose, until it is in the right range, via blood retesting. That's why some people (I was one of them) feel no difference at all for a while because you simply break even until you get the right amount in you that is adequate to restore metabolism in the body completely.

It's too bad there are so many of these crazy issues that can affect our treatment but all we can do, is the best we can!

QUESTION FIFTY-TWO

Should I be Firm in Requesting Thyroid Blood Testing?

My reply on a forum Re: "Being Firm in Requesting Thyroid Blood Testing".---

All the symptoms you describe sound like classic hypothyroid symptoms, in fact it is almost like reading a list from a medical site! The cysts you refer-to are probably "nodules" (small benign tumors in the gland) but your Dr. will need to determine this for sure. Nodules and goiters (thyroid enlargement and bumps), are common with autoimmune thyroid disease, which is the most common cause of hypothyroidism (low thyroid function). It is also called "Hashimoto's Thyroiditis".

Request (firmly) that your Dr. order a thyroid panel with "thyroid antibodies" tests along with it. I say to be firm in requesting these because he is working for you, not the other way around and your health is an important possession, worthy of through evaluation. I'm not telling you to be rude but do be firm because you are your own advocate in getting proper care.

Eighty-Seven Thyroid Disease Questions Answered!

YES, Dr.s will sometimes act arrogant towards patients and think it is ridiculous for them to suggest a test etc... but if one is too reluctant to see the importance of through evaluation, it may be time for a new Dr. (2nd opinion). It is your body and you have rights, as a patient to protect your life and ability to continue with your livelihood and support of your family. Also make sure they give you photo-copies of all lab results because YOU PAY FOR THEM and they are obliged by "HIPPA law" to provide them upon your request (this may require signing a release). This way, it will help you in case you want to research the results online or share them with others, like those of us at fellow-patient forums.

I am a Hashimoto's – hypothyroidism patient, as are many on this forum.

QUESTION FIFTY-THREE

Is there a Relationship of TSH and Thyroid Antibodies to Hypothyroid Symptoms?

My forum comment Re: "Relationship of TSH and Thyroid Antibodies to Hypothyroid Symptoms".---

First, that TSH reading (3.9) is actually high for a hypothyroid patient on thyroid replacement medication. Every reputable site I have ever looked at to see what recommendations were for TSH levels in patients on replacement hormone medication said it should be between 1.0 to 2.0 but they also say that some patients only have relief of symptoms when theirs is less than 1.0. You can actually get down to 0.35 and not yet be in hyperthyroidism/overactive territory. I've had mine down to 0.45 and had no hyper type symptoms at all, in fact I still had some hypothyroid symptoms until mine was lowered/suppressed even more with an increased dose (my T4 and T3 would remain in normal range).

The "American Association of Clinical Endocrinologists" came out with NEW GUIDELINES for TSH levels in 2002 and most labs have not re-adjusted their ranges as yet.

Eighty-Seven Thyroid Disease Questions Answered!

This organization which is the most reliable source for endocrinology standards (thyroid is in this category), issued the new guidelines for TSH as being "0.3 to 3.0" and stated that anyone with a TSH of 3.0 is suspect for hypothyroidism. With yours being 3.9, you could easily still be experiencing hypothyroid symptoms! If you'll do a search and put in the key words "New TSH standards", you'll find these new guidelines. Your Microsomal antibodies also sound very high but I'm not familiar with that name and is likely the same as the TPO antibodies (anti-thyroidperoxidase). Usually the other ones they check are called the anti-thyroglobulin – abbreviated "TG" (which you noted was normal) along with the TPO ones. Did the microsomal one have a reference range? I can almost guarantee you that the microsomal level/result you posted (in the 100s) is HIGH! But, I would like to see the normal values range. Usually a range will look like this: "<40" or something to that effect, meaning your antibodies should be that number or less. That's the same range my lab had on the antithyroidperoxidase one, so that reading you reported is very high in comparison to that type of range! Some people with Hashimoto's thyroiditis have only one or the other that's high (positive) and some have both of them high.

Eighty-Seven Thyroid Disease Questions Answered!

It's my understanding that the TPO one is even more important than the TG one.

I don't know a great deal about the ANA (anti-nuclear antibodies) test, as it relates to thyroid disease except that mine was negative when I had it tested (I believe the test is to detect "systemic" - body wide autoimmunity). Thyroid antibodies are suppose to go down over time with thyroid hormone medication but some medical sites I have read/searched, said that it can take years for this to occur. I feel high antibodies in autoimmune hypothyroid disease, can cause symptoms as much as low hormone levels can and there are medical studies confirming this fact.

QUESTION FIFTY-FOUR

Can Thyroid Antibodies Cause Chronic Hives?

My forum post regarding "Thyroid Antibodies can Cause Chronic Hives".---

You don't see hives mentioned on very many medical sites but high level (positive) thyroid antibodies can cause them.

The reason I searched about this is because I came down with severe hives just before being diagnosed with Hashimoto's Disease but I did not make the connection until two years later, when I found mention of it happening with Hashimoto's thyroiditis, on medical research sources. I had NEVER had hives before and not since being treated for hypothyroidism but they are always an immune system reaction (i.e. from allergies or antibodies) or in response to tremendous stress (traumatic or chronic). I agree that they should run thyroid panel blood tests for your son, due to his unexplainable hives - also called "chronic urticaria" and keep blood testing any areas of suspicion until an answer is found for what is causing them. My "Eos"(eosinophils) were also flagged "high" when blood testing was ordered to find my Hashimoto's/hypothyroidism thyroid disorder, which indicated an allergy, which may have also contributed to my hives.

QUESTION FIFTY-FIVE

Are there any Basic Questions New Thyroid Patients should ask Doctors?

My forum post Re: "Basic Questions New Thyroid Patients should Ask Doctors".---

Your diagnosis of hypothyroidism is due to your TSH being elevated and as far as the T-4 level, I would need to see the range the lab used as a reference, in order to comment on it. Your TSH though is definitely elevated above normal because most labs have a normal values range of about 0.5 to 5.0. The reason TSH elevates is because your thyroid is under active and TSH (Thyroid Stimulating Hormone), is trying to get your low functioning thyroid to produce more hormone, as your levels have begun to drop. Did they check your thyroid antibody levels? This would be the Anti-Thyroglobulin and Anti-Thyroperoxidase Antibodies. These two tests are to see if autoimmune disease of the thyroid is causing the hypothyroidism. There are other causes, so these tests would be helpful if you have not already been ordered them. Have they or are they going to place you on thyroid hormone replacement medication?

Have they mentioned you having a goiter or nodule (tumor in your gland)? These are questions you might ask your doctor if he has not already gone over these issues with you.

Also, a really good information source is the thyroid.about.com website (by: Mary Shomon) but you'll get good research info by simply going to a search engine and putting in key words like "hypothyroidism, hashimoto's thyroiditis, thyroid disorders", etc... . Also make sure you get your own copies of every test you have done. You pay for them and it's your right by law to obtain them. This way, it will help you with research you do and questions you ask of other patients like us, at this forum. If you have your lab report, post for us, all the readings on it, including the reference ranges and we might be able to comment more.

QUESTION FIFTY-SIX

When are Antidepressants needed by Treated Thyroid Patients?

From my forum post Re: "When Antidepressants are Needed by Treated Thyroid Patients".---

The people on this forum always give such good advice! I too am a Hashimoto's/Hypothyroidism sufferer and Dr.s were constantly trying to put me on antidepressants, in fact the first Dr. I visited suggested them and I went ahead and took them for a few months then had to stop them slowly/gradually because my untreated thyroid disease worsened! I then realized even when I did finally get tested for thyroid disease and was placed on medication/treatment for it, that it would be hard to distinguish the side effects of an antidepressant from unrelieved thyroid symptoms, had I continued them.

Please don't take this as a recommendation to stop your antidepressant. This should NEVER be done apart from doctor-supervision. If you are getting thyroid treatment simultaneously with the antidepressant, this might work for you, if both are needed. I would however, read thoroughly, the drug-insert that came with the antidepressant or go online and search "side effects of (your drugs name)". Also, never stop taking an antidepressant suddenly. These have to be weaned off of, very gradually and with professional medical supervision. ALSO, you can have both hyperthyroid and hypothyroid symptoms at the same time.

In fact there is an article on this by same title "Can I Be Hypothyroid and Hyperthyroid at The Same Time?" (By: Mary Shomon), just go to a search engine and put these search-words in and I bet it'll pop up and be very informative in regard to your case of having the symptoms of both.

Lastly, have they tested your thyroid antibody levels? If not, you should consider requesting them.

QUESTION FIFTY-SEVEN

Are Mood Disorders Common with Thyroid Disease?

My forum post Re: "Mood Disorders are Common with Thyroid Disease".---

I hope you finally get an attentive, compassionate Dr. this time. Most of us have been through a few that weren't very caring. You never know when a new, more specialized Dr. might have much better revelations for you. The "Free T-3 and Free T-4" I have heard, are the best thyroid hormones to have done.

Eighty-Seven Thyroid Disease Questions Answered!

This as opposed to just T-3 and T-4, which are also called by names such as "Total T-4, Thyroxin", etc... The ones with the word "Free" in front of them, measure the free, unbound hormone levels, which informed doctors say are the best to get tested, for superior accuracy.

If they try to indicate that you're a mental case, set them straight! Low mood and anxiety commonly co-exist with thyroid disorders and they should know this but sometimes they try to convince patients that their symptoms are psycho-somatic (emotionally caused). Research I've done states that only about 20% of Major Depression sufferers have severe fatigue and serious joint pain is not as common with emotional problems as they would like us to think (body aches are usually vague with mood disorders but more prominent with physical diseases).

I asked several people with severe depression but no thyroid disease, if they had joint aches with their mood disorder and they didn't even know what I was talking about.

My belief is that so many Dr.s, for so many years have treated medical conditions like thyroid disease, with antidepressants (which won't work, unless the disease is treated as well), that they really do believe joint swelling, chronic fatigue etc... are all emotional manifestations. I hope this trend will someday stop, so that needed diagnoses and treatments can be received by more people needing them!

QUESTION FIFTY-EIGHT

What is the Purpose of Thyroid Antibody Testing?

A FORUM POST I MADE Re: "The Purpose of Thyroid Antibody Testing".---

The thyroid antibodies test is to see if your hypothyroidism is caused by autoimmune disease (Hashimoto's) or in the case of hyperthyroidism, if it is caused by Grave's disease. Autoimmune disease occurs when your body produces antibodies against an organ/gland, as if it is an intruder. Normally antibodies attack true invaders such as viruses and germs etc... but for some reason the body recognizes part of itself as an invader.

Dr.s don't yet know the reason this happens but in the case of the thyroid, it causes tissue destruction that is irreversible, which results in reduced ability for it to produce adequate hormone levels (hypothyroidism). Don't let this scare you because it is the most common cause of hypothyroidism in industrialized countries. This is the kind I have. My Anti-Thyroglobulins ABs were "537" (normal range was <35) and my Anti-Thyroperoxidase ABs were "120" (normal being <40), so elevated levels of these are how they determine if you have Hashimoto's thyroiditis (named after the Japanese Dr. who discovered it in 1912).

Another reason they check for thyroid antibodies is because autoimmune diseases many times run together, in fact Hashimoto's and Autoimmune Adrenal Insufficiency (Addison's Disease) can co-exist. The Dr. probably wants to see if you could possibly have "Schmidt's Syndrome" (Hypothyroid and Addison's disease, combined) or a polyglandular disease of another kind. I hope you don't have one of these combination disorders but there are treatments for them that keep people running normal by replacing any needed hormones that are low.

For low thyroid, they give you thyroid hormone replacement and for low adrenal they usually give you hydrocortisone and/or fludrocortisone.

QUESTION FIFTY-NINE

Any Advice Regarding Hypothyroid Treatment and Adrenal Fatigue?

From my forum post Re: "Hypothyroid Treatment and Adrenal Fatigue".---

It's seems I have something in common with so many people on this forum. I too felt I had adrenal insufficiency along with my Hashimoto's/Hypothyroidism because I had worsened hypothyroid symptoms after starting my thyroid hormone replacement medication. I had read that this can happen if you have a degree of low-adrenal function and you don't treat it before starting thyroid medication. So, I started out by doing home saliva-tests offered by Great Smokey Mountain Diagnostic Labs, Inc., who market cortisol/DHEA adrenal hormone tests under the name "BodyBalance StressChek".

The first one I had done showed low-normal cortisol, so I did a second one a few months later and it showed clinically low levels of cortisol (the major stress/adrenal hormone).

I took these labs to my Dr. and he had me do an ACTH Stimulation test (designed to detect full-blown adrenal insufficiency). I passed the test, so he said it wasn't "Addison's Disease" (true adrenal gland disease) however, there are secondary forms of adrenal insufficiency that cause low cortisol levels, which he seemed to not know about. Anyway, I also did a 24-hour urinary cortisol test which also came out very low (range for adult males was <119, mine was "10.7"). I truly believe my cortisol levels dropped even further when I started my thyroid medication.

I can guarantee that your better informed Dr. is testing you because of concern your adrenal insufficiency might be worsened if not treated along with your hypothyroidism, if it does happen to also be low. Some medical sites state that Hashimoto's and adrenal insufficiency often co-exist, due to the autoimmune process that can be common with both.

They actually have a name for it "Schmidt's Disease" and if you have several low functioning glands, including pancreas (diabetes) and pernicious anemia, they call it "Polyglandular Autoimmune Disease II". I hope they find yours to only be a mild secondary adrenal insufficiency. Your Dr. is wise in checking for this. Most Dr.s don't test for comorbid adrenal dysfunction even though it is even recommended in the Physicians Desk Reference, that adrenal hormones need checked BEFORE thyroid hormone is administered in a patient. A lot of Dr.s have no idea about these things, which is a bit scary but it sounds like you have a good one who has your best interests at heart!

One more thing to keep in mind is that low-normal thyroid hormones and HIGH-normal TSH readings are sometimes not really normal especially if you have elevated (positive) thyroid antibodies levels. Example: TSH can be in a range of 0.5 to 5.0 but if your result is "4.9" it is well worth further observation. Example 2: If free T-3 is in a range of 2.4 to 4.5 and yours is "2.5" it is worth further observation. When I was diagnosed hypothyroid, my TSH was "8.3" but all other hormones were in low-normal.

Eighty-Seven Thyroid Disease Questions Answered!

I later found out that my thyroid antibodies were highly elevated and was why I had full-blown symptoms. I did also have a low "T-3 Uptake" but they still called it "sub-Clinical" hypothyroidism. Hormones can fluctuate during the autoimmune attack with Hashimoto's thyroiditis (the type I have).

QUESTION SIXTY

When is it Important to Determine the Cause of Hypothyroidism?

From my forum post Re: "Determining the Cause of Hypothyroidism".---

That is for sure an elevated TSH level (10.0 and above) because most labs have a range of about 0.5 to 5.0. My TSH at the time I was diagnosed hypothyroid was "8.3" and I also had a T-3 Uptake flagged "low". If they didn't do more tests than this in your case (TSH only), I'm willing to bet they probably will at some point.

Eighty-Seven Thyroid Disease Questions Answered!

Make sure you tell them you want a "thyroid antibodies" panel and don't let them talk you out of it! This test will tell you if the hypothyroidism is due to autoimmune disease or if negative, that it's possibly another reason.

My antibodies were as follows on mine:

Anti-thyroglobulin "537" (normal being <40)

Anti-thyroperoxidase "120" (normal being <35).

Dr.s are not always as knowledgeable about thyroid disorders as you might think and will tell you it doesn't matter what's causing the hypothyroidism. However, it does matter because Hashimoto's Thyroiditis is an autoimmune disease and the most common cause of hypothyroidism in industrialized countries.

Autoimmune Disease needs close monitoring because you are susceptible to other autoimmune diseases when one is present. It can also cause goiter (thyroid enlargement) and nodules (thyroid gland tumors).

These are usually easily manageable with thyroid hormone replacement medication which also helps control your hypothyroid symptoms. Let us know about future labs you have done, for more comments when we are able to provide them. You might also do some search engine research. Just put in key words like "hypothyroidism, Hashimoto's Disease", etc... . There is also an informative sight at www.thyroid.about.com published by Thyroid Patient Advocate – Mary Shomon.

SECTION FIVE:
Questions and Answers SIXTY-ONE through SEVENTY-FIVE

QUESTION SIXTY-ONE

Can one have both Hypothyroid and Hyperthyroid Symptoms?

From my forum post Re: "Having both Hypothyroid and Hyperthyroid Symptoms".---

Your heart palpitations and lack of weight gain sounds more in the hyperthyroidism category, however, they most likely came to the hypothyroidism conclusion because of lab results. Did you have blood tests? If so, do you know what your results and the reference ranges were? If they did not provide you a copy of your lab work, I would request one because you pay for these and should be given a copy of all labs done. If you can get these, get back on this forum and tell us what they were and we might be able to comment on them.

One of the more important tests to diagnose Hashimoto's Thyroiditis (the most common cause of hypothyroidism) are the "Thyroid Antibodies Tests". This usually includes the anti-thyroglobulin and anti-thyroperoxidase antibodies. There are also antibodies that help diagnose Graves Disease (autoimmune hyperthyroidism) from other types of thyroid disorders (thyroid stimulating immunoglobulin) but they look at the antibodies in conjunction with thyroid hormone levels. If the hormones are low along with antibodies being elevated, it is certain to be autoimmune hypothyroidism.

Another important thing to remember though, is that with Hashimoto's (autoimmune hypothyroid), you can swing back and forth between hypo and hyper because the antibody attack against your thyroid (autoimmune thyroiditis), will sometimes actually cause the thyroid to overproduce hormone (intermittent hyperthyroidism) in it's attempt to fight off the attack but it will always return back to a hypothyroid state and will eventually remain so, progressively once enough thyroid tissue has been permanently destroyed by the autoimmune process.

This may be why you are having both hyper and hypo symptoms almost simultaneously. I hope this helps, in the mean time, shoot us those lab readings if you can and want to, because most of us out hereon the forum, are very familiar with those due to seeing so many of our own.

QUESTION SIXTY-TWO

Do you know anything about the Evaluation of Thyroid Nodules?

From a forum post I made Re: "The Evaluation of thyroid Nodules".---

Only a very small percent of nodules are cancerous and if they already told you this is not a concern, they are probably certain. They can actually tell what kind of nodule you have by feeling (palpating) it. The size and firmness etc... tells them a lot about the type nodule you have. I think if you go to the new specialist you mentioned being referred to, I would only have it removed if they believe it needs to be.

I know it is very hard to accept something being in your body like this, that's causing a problem but I'm not so sure removal of the nodule would stop the autoimmune process. Some researchers believe nodules are simply a symptom of a problem that's deeper inside the thyroid. Try to be patient (easier said than done) because it is good that they are taking time to thoroughly evaluate the best treatment possible for you. In the mean time, shoot us any questions that might come up. We may have helpful opinions or sometimes we might not know anything beyond very basic information but it always helps to communicate with other fellow-patient sufferers.

QUESTION SIXTY-THREE

Are there Thyroid Antibodies that cause Hypothyroid and Hyperthyroid Symptoms?

From a forum post I made, Re: "Thyroid Antibodies causing Hypothyroid and Hyperthyroid Symptoms".---

Eighty-Seven Thyroid Disease Questions Answered!

First, a person with thyroid antibodies can most certainly have thyroid symptoms of both hyperthyroidism and hypothyroidism. If your Dr. doesn't seem to know this, you might think about a new Dr. (but I'm sure he/she does). Your description of symptoms, including the eye irritation are classic for thyroid disorder. It is true that sometimes a Dr.s doesn't know when to treat and it is a difficult decision for them when you are totting back and forth between hypothyroid and hyperthyroid sumptoms but this is a common happening when you have autoimmune thyroid disease. If what you have is Hashimoto's Thyroiditis, the hyper times will eventually stop happening because your thyroid will begin to fizzle-out. It actually becomes damaged by the auto-antibodies attacking and it loses its ability to produce adequate levels of thyroid hormone and you'll become permanently "hypothyroid". At that time, they will be able to see this on your hormone blood level tests.

Your TSH which is probably in normal range only for now, will become elevated (the pituitary hormone that kick-starts your thyroid to produce) and your other thyroid hormones will begin to drop to low levels.

Usually, as soon as they see the TSH elevate, they'll treat you with replacement thyroid hormone because you also have antibodies and the hormone will actually shrink any existing goiters or nodules. Unless they are the type that need further attention and only your Dr. can determine this.

The medication will also relieve your "hypothyroid" symptoms, although some of us have lingering symptoms such as fatigue and joint aches. Your weight loss, followed by weight gain also have to do with your condition. You could on the other hand, have Graves' Disease which is also autoimmune but causes only hyperthyroidism and not the hypothyroid type symptoms you have occurring with yours. Graves can be temporary in some cases whereas Hashimoto's Disease is almost always permanent. With Graves', they sometimes kill-off the thyroid gland (ablation) with radio-active iodine because the hyperthyroid state causes some people, serious heart and blood pressure problems. Once they kill off a Graves' thyroid, that person has to take thyroid replacement medication afterward, just like hypothyroid people do.

Eighty-Seven Thyroid Disease Questions Answered!

I've been in your place and needed answers badly, so wanted to give you the best summation of thyroid disorders that I could.

QUESTION SIXTY-FOUR

Any Association between Thyroid Disease and Orthostatic Hypotension?

Derived from a forum post I made Re: "Thyroid Disease and Orthostatic Hypotension".---

I too have had many times of wondering when my thyroid-related symptoms will all get significant under control (as you also expressed in your post). I too had increased vision problems after getting Hashimoto's thyroiditis (possibly coincidental and not part of the disease). That was interesting, your mention of having to stand in one spot until the orthostatic intolerance passed, when you first stand up (symptoms of sudden blood pressure drop).

I've had people see me do this, plus I would steady myself with a hand on the wall and they'd say "what's wrong?" and I'd say "just another dizzy spell from standing up!" This is also called Orthostatic Hypotension" (O.I.) and is a form of "dysautonomia", meaning an imbalance in the automonic nervous system (also called "the involuntary nervous system"). This is the part of the N.S. that regulates blood pressure, heart rate etc... .

Dysautonomia sometimes co-exists with autoimmune diseases. O. I. is not supposed to be harmful or dangerous unless you fall down from it. They only recommend treatment for it when it is bad enough that you actually pass out from it. All I know is that it sure is a bummer! One last mention of this condition is that researchers have found O.I. to be a common component of both Chronic Fatigue Syndrome and fibromyalgia, which are also now recognized as being autoimmune related diseases by some medical researchers.

QUESTION SIXTY-FIVE

Should a Treated Hypothyroid Patient be Struggling with Weight Gain?

The post following, was a reply on a thyroid forum I made to a "Treated Hypothyroid Patient Struggling with Weight Gain" and difficulty losing weight.---

You posted a reply to my question about joint aches. I want to reply to yours as well. I'm a male, however, I too have an incredible time trying to lose weight since having Hashimoto's/Hypothyroidism.

I wanted to do an overall improvement in all areas, including weight, so that I could get ahead of this thing but instead of losing, I've actually gained since being on thyroid hormone replacement medication. I too am not morbidly obese but moderately overweight. Please stay encouraged as much as possible, you have friends out here in the same mess you're in. I don't know if it's true because there are so many opinions out there in the medical but some say that once the thyroid completely atrophies (dies off from disease), people then see improvements.

Eighty-Seven Thyroid Disease Questions Answered!

The antibody levels that cause hypothyroidism in most cases, in industrialized countries, then begin to significantly decrease. I hope it's true but regardless, please hang in there and keep researching because you'll find a good nugget of knowledge once in a while and suggestions that will help. Put them all together at some point and you might have a completed puzzle.

QUESTION SIXTY-SIX

Are there some Uninformed Doctors Treating Thyroid Diseases?

The following is derived from a thyroid support forum post I made in the year 2005 regarding "Uninformed Doctors Treating Thyroid Diseases".---

The more I read others comments, the more amazed I become! I too am terribly frustrated with doctors (it took me five to get diagnosed). They are overbooked and burned-out and worse than that, they are often totally lacking compassion.

Eighty-Seven Thyroid Disease Questions Answered!

I too was diagnosed as a mental case at first and placed on an antidepressant, Xanax and a beta-blocker. These made my untreated thyroid much worse! Some people have not yet understood that most Dr.s today are very uninformed about thyroid disorders. For example, you'll hear a Dr. say: "Only a TSH test is necessary to diagnose thyroid imbalance." What's strange about that opinion is the fact that Graves Disease and Hashimoto's thyroiditis both can manifest with "normal TSH" levels, with the actual thyroid hormones being affected independently of the TSH level (because of thyroid antibodies).

ALSO, a person can have symptoms even with all hormones in normal range, if antibody levels remain high because and I quote from many reputable sites: "High antibody levels will cause reduced ability for thyroid hormones to bind to receptors, resulting in hypothyroid symptoms even while levels are within normal range."

WE PATIENTS should not have to do Dr.s jobs! But since this uninformed trend is going on with some Dr.s (but not all of them), we better keep researching and sharing research with one another.

QUESTION SIXTY-SEVEN

Can Joint Pain occur with Treated Hypothyroidism?

Article derived from a forum post I made in year 2005, regarding "Joint Pain with Treated Hypothyroidism".---

Thanks so much ladies for your input, that is truly amazing and I have a feeling it is a common problem with Hashimoto's thyroiditis sufferers.

You mentioned joint aches worse with the thyroid hormone replacement medication. Strange you should say that, I often comment to my wife, that my joint aches became much worse with the medication and she remembers this too.

Back when I had been on medication only a few months, I got discouraged and so I did a search, using key words "reasons thyroid replacement medication may have adverse effects", or something to that effect and it took me to sights stating "untreated adrenal cortical insufficiency may become worse after starting thyroid medication", in fact ALL BRANDS of thyroid medication have this warning in their literature.

Eighty-Seven Thyroid Disease Questions Answered!

So, I searched "symptoms of adrenal insufficiency" and there listed, were the same symptoms for hypothyroid, including fatigue (Which I also still have - do you?) and the sites also listed joint pain for adrenal disorders, etc...

This prompted me to order a home Stress Hormone Test from GSMDL, Inc. and over the past year, I have done 4 of these and each time, my cortisol (the major stress hormone) was low-normal, borderline-low and even clinically-low on one of them. I've also found sites stating that 25% of Hashimoto's patients develop other problems, such as adrenal insufficiency, anemia (I was borderline) and diabetes (I was borderline on this too).

It's funny how the typical Dr. will not tell you these things. Have you ladies read Mary Shomon's book "Living Well with Autoimmune Disease"? I highly recommend it if not. Mary relates experiencing a time of unrelieved symptoms in her book even while on thyroid replacement (she has Hashimoto's hypothyroidism) so I knew I related well to her problem but I wanted to hear from others on this too.

QUESTION SIXTY-EIGHT

Can you share Symptom Problems you experienced with Hypothyroid Treatment?

The following article is derived from a post I made on a thyroid patient support forum in 2005. The post reveals the type "Symptom Problems I Experienced with my Hypothyroid Treatment".---

I'm an age-42 man (this year of 2005) with Hashimoto's thyroiditis and was wondering if any of you out there with the same, have joint pain even though on medication?

I have already been tested for RA Factor, Uric Acid, ANA, ESR possibilities but all were negative. After being on thyroid medication for two years and getting my TSH in good range "1.0" and my other thyroid hormones in the upper half of the ranges, I asked for the antibodies tests because none of the five Dr.s I've gone to, for getting proper treatment, would suggest one. My Anti-thyroglobulin ABs were "537" (normal being <40) and my Anti-Peroxidase ABs were "120" (normal being <35).

Eighty-Seven Thyroid Disease Questions Answered!

When I originally was diagnosed hypothyroid, my TSH was "8.3" (moderately high) and the other abnormal was a T-3 Uptake, flagged "low". Other than this, labs were in lower half of normal ranges. The Dr.s claimed this was only "sub-clinical Hypothyroidism" however, this part I now know was BALONEY (excuse my bluntness)! With Hashmoto's, TSH and other levels can fluctuate! ANYWAY, to sum up my question, do you guys/gals believe HIGH ANTIBODY LEVELS, can perpetuate symptoms, even while on thyroid hormone replacement? AND, do any of you have joint pain even on treatment? My joint pain is almost all upper body, cervical spine, shoulders and collar bones but occasionally my feet ache in the arches of them too.

QUESTION SIXTY-NINE

Natural Supplements for Autoimmune Hypothyroidism?

There are natural ways to compliment or what you might call "supplementing" your hypothyroid therapy but none of these are a substitute for thyroid hormone replacement therapy.

Eighty-Seven Thyroid Disease Questions Answered!

For example, a healthy diet, exercise and healthy supplements (i.e. vitamins and safe, well-researched herbals containing no-iodine) can help, being careful to take those that contain calcium or iron, about six hours apart from thyroid hormone dose. I also believe-in running any supplements past a person's treating doctor, to help determine their safety.

As far as something that can substitute thyroid hormone replacement, there simply is nothing that can do this because the body absolutely requires it. It is also important that you are assured by your doctor that your treatment has been best-possible optimized. He can do this by going over your follow-up blood retests showing where your thyroid hormone levels are. There are medical studies published by the U.S.-NIH (PubMed) stating that "selenium" supplementation can reduce antibody levels and activity (i.e. inflammation and swelling) in cases of autoimmune hypothyroidism.

Autoimmunity of any kind is a strange phenomenon that medical research is trying to understand more, as they conduct further research. Some sources state that autoimmunity is caused by an overactive immune system.

Eighty-Seven Thyroid Disease Questions Answered!

QUOTE: "People with lupus have an overactive immune system." from MedicineNet.com - By the site Medical Editor: William C. Shiel Jr., MD, FACP, FACR is an example of this opinion.

I also feel in some people, diseases of autoimmunity can point-to "immune deficiency" because I for example have autoimmune thyroid disease - Hashimoto's thyroiditis but I also have immune deficiency in other areas. I have CFS (Chronic Fatigue Syndrome) co-morbid to thyroid autoimmunity and mild asthma which both point-to immune deficiency. It's almost as if in some patients, their immune system contradicts itself (overactive and under-active simultaneously) and is why it's so important to have a good doctor to evaluate what's needed in each autoimmune disease patient.

QUESTION SEVENTY

Can TSH at "7.0" Represent Hypothyroidism?

Many blood testing labs are now setting their high-normal cut-off value for TSH at about 4.5, so a reading of 7.0 is elevated.

TSH rises above normal with hypothyroidism (under-active thyroid). If your thyroid hormone levels are not falling below normal at the same time TSH is rising, you may only have sub-clinical hypothyroidism but only your doctor can tell you for sure. Regardless, if you need treated, it simply requires that your doctor prescribe a daily dose of a thyroid hormone replacement drug. Over time, the dose will correct your low metabolism by getting your thyroid hormones back to euthroid level (normal).

Hypothyroidism can develop before the T3 and/or T4 fall below normal values. Some people see TSH rise to between 10.0 and 15.0 and thyroid hormones are still within normal range. A "7.0" TSH is elevated according to all lab ranges for it that I have seen because highest normal averages about "5.0" at many labs but can be as high as 6.0 at a few of them. Some labs place highest-normal TSH at 4.0 and some experts even believe readings above 3.0 indicate developing hypothyroidism. In my opinion a 7.0 reading merits follow up every few months by repeat blood testing despite normal T3 and T4 levels.

QUESTION SEVENTY-ONE

What is the Goal of Thyroid Hormone Replacement?

The goal of thyroid hormone replacement is to suppress the TSH level (pituitary hormone) and to elevate the T4 and T3 to mid-range or above. A blood TSH level over "10.0" indicates overt (full blown) hypothyroidism. TSH elevates with hypothyroidism, while the thyroid hormones (T4 & T3) decrease to abnormally low levels. The average normal value at blood testing labs for TSH is roughly 0.4 to 4.5 and your thyroid dose will need to get your TSH back down into this normal values range. Some doctors have a goal of suppressing TSH down to between "1.0 and 2.0" to successfully resolve hypothyroid symptoms of fatigue, weight gain, dry skin, constipation, etc...

Thyroid hormone replacement medications are designed to replace the low level no longer being supplied by the thyroid gland or "hypothyroidism" (under active). This condition causes a slowing of the metabolism which means fuels coming into the body (i.e. food and oxygen) are burned/used at a slower rate.

Eighty-Seven Thyroid Disease Questions Answered!

By administering thyroid hormone therapy - dosed to a proper level, the metabolism is brought back up to normal speed.

If once a proper dose level is reached and even more hormone is added (unnecessary dose increase - over treatment) the metabolism then becomes abnormally sped-up. This would be referred to as dose induced "thyrotoxicity" (hyperthyroidism-overactive). An overactive thyroid gland or thyrotoxicity from whatever cause (i.e. Graves' disease, thyroid hormone drug overdosing, hot nodules in the thyroid gland, etc...), will typically cause weight loss. One reason for this is because food passes through the body too quickly for nutrients to be absorbed or for fat to be stored in the body. This is also why diarrhea is a common symptom listed for hyperthyroidism.

QUESTION SEVENTY-TWO

Can Goiter cause Thyroid Swelling on One Side?

Your isthmus (middle portion of the thyroid) is centered in the gland and the two lobes (one on each side) extend upward and are attached to the Adams apple via connecting cartilage (the Adams apple itself is cartilage). It is a butterfly-shaped gland, located just below the Adams apple in the front-middle of the neck.

When a goiter (swelling) begins, it can affect only one lobe and a lobe can be affected by a "thyroid nodule" causing it to protrude as well. If both goiter and nodule are present, they refer to it as a "nodular goiter".

Your doctor can palpate your gland (feel with fingertips) to see if he detects a nodule and whether if feels firm or not. From there he would likely order a thyroid ultrasound and/or a thyroid uptake scan (radioactive iodine dose, followed by radiological imaging).

If a thyroid nodule is found and is of a large size or it appears solid, a thyroid tissue biopsy might follow. This is what is also referred to as a "Fine Needle Aspiration" to make sure no cancer cells are present.

If no nodules are found, you may simply be experiencing thyroid autoimmunity with resulting inflammation which will eventually lead to hypothyroidism (low functioning) and the goiter may shrink once you're placed on thyroid hormone replacement - once needed.

If you have a mild, temporary goiter which can occur with respiratory viruses, it will resolve over a few weeks time. Your doctor can better determine the cause of the swollen thyroid lobe or even determine that the swelling is not in your thyroid but rather in a lymph node located near the thyroid gland.

QUESTION SEVENTY-THREE

Why Would TSH be Low but Throxine (T4) Normal?

This question I respond-to following below, was asked by someone who had a low TSH blood result ("0.287") but a normal T4 (thyroxine level):
- - -

A result on TSH of 0.287 is only very slightly below the lowest-normal cut-off value of "0.3". This type result would merit follow up, to make sure it is not continuing to drop because a flagged-low TSH usually represents hyperthyroidism (overactive thyroid). If a lab has "0.25" as the low normal reference range, yours would still be within normal but being near borderline, would still merit a repeat blood test within a few months to see if it has dropped further. Testing both the T3 and T4 thyroid hormone levels might be wise as well and tests for thyroid antibodies - the immune cells that cause autoimmune thyroid disease.

Some people have TSH levels that do not accurately reflect their thyroid hormone levels and I'm one of them.

Eighty-Seven Thyroid Disease Questions Answered!

As a treated hypothyroid patient (under-active thyroid gland), my TSH has to be suppressed to below-normal levels, to get my thyroxine (T4) and my T3 levels up to at least mid-range. TSH normally elevates with hypothyroidism and usually goes low with hyperthyroidism (overactive).

Another possibility is that you have a pituitary gland problem - the one that sends TSH to the thyroid, causing it to release proper amounts of hormone. If there is a small tumor in the pituitary it can cause it to be sluggish in sending enough TSH, which is referred-to as "hypopituitarism". If this is the case, your thyroxine may have been normal-range but in the "low-normal". Over time, if it is your pituitary is failing to send adequate amounts of TSH to stimulate the thyroid gland, you'll eventually develop "Central Hypothyroidism" (failure of the central command - brain center).

The third possibility is that you are very early into the onset of hyperthyroidism and your TSH is starting to go lower as your thyroxine level rises. Over time, the thyroxine will go outside of the normal values (flagged high) if this is the case.

Graves' disease is the most common cause of hyperthyroidism, so you may need to be tested for "thyroid antibodies" that cause the disease - referred to as "Thyroid Stimulating Immunoglobulin". In my opinion your TSH and thyroxine levels merit follow up blood retesting as well, within two or three months, so you should discuss this with your doctor.

QUESTION SEVENTY-FOUR

Can Elevated Thyroid Hormone Levels cause Anxiety?

Anxiety, nervousness and panic attacks are listed commonly for hyperthyroid conditions (overactive thyroid), including Graves' disease (autoimmune caused) and a condition called "Hashitoxicosis" which can occur, just before a person begins to experience hypothyroidism (under active thyroid).

When a goiter (thyroid swelling) occurs with hyperthyroidism, it is called a "toxic diffuse goiter".

If small tumor-like growths develop in the gland, that causes it to produce excessive amounts of hormone, they are called "hot nodules". Someone being treated for hypothyroidism with thyroid hormone replacement, can develop anxiety symptoms as well if their dose is too high, which is called "thyrotoxicity".

All of these hyperthyroid conditions have potential to cause anxiety symptoms and if you do a search using "hyperthyroid symptoms" as a term with a search engine, this anxiety will come up often as part of the symptom-complex. Yes, thyroid imbalance can most-definitely manifest with anxiety symptoms, among others.

QUESTION SEVENTY-FIVE

Can Hyperthyroidism be resolved with Drug Treatment Only?

The answer that follows below, was to a question posted to me by a hyperthyroid patient who was treated with an anti-thyroid drug only (NeoMercazole) and afterward they were placed on thyroid hormone replacement (Eltroxin) for hypothyroidism. It is actually rare for hyperthyroid cases to not require destruction or removal of the thyroid gland and is one of several points I made in my comments to them that follow. ---

NeoMercazole is an antithyroid medication that slows thyroid hormone production in an overactive gland. With your hyperthyroidism resolving with this medication and not also requiring thyroid removal, it may have been a rare case in which Graves' disease (autoimmune caused hyperthyroidism) resolved without further treatment. It may also be that your case was actually that of Hashimoto's thyroiditis (autoimmune caused hypothyroidism) which can first present with a phase of hyperthyroidism - "Hashitoxicosis".

Your doctor could order tests for Anti-TPO and anti-TG antibodies and if one or both are positive, Hashimoto's would be a strong possibility. A tissue biopsy called an "FNA" (Fine Needle Aspiration) and a thyroid ultrasound would help confirm this as well, plus the latter one can help detect whether any thyroid nodules are present. The type called "hot nodules" can also be a cause of hyperthyroidism.

Eltroxin is a thyroid hormone replacement drug and many Thyroid Specialists and Endocrinologists suggest getting the TSH level (a blood hormone level most often used to monitor thyroid hormone replacement), suppressed down to between "1.0 and 2.0" to better optimized relief of hypothyroid symptoms (like fatigue). Some use "1.0" as their target treatment goal. These are things you might consider discussing with your doctor, to better understand your case.

SECTION SIX:
Questions and Answers SEVENTY-SIX through EIGHTY-SEVEN

QUESTION SEVENTY-SIX

Do Thyroid Antibodies Continue with Hypothyroid Therapy?

Hashimoto's is a lifelong autoimmune thyroiditis and the resulting hypothyroidism it causes, requires permanent treatment as well. Some people diagnosed with underactive thyroid glands are not afterward tested for causes of it but the most common cause in industrialized countries like the UK and US, is Hashimoto's. Treating-doctors vary in how often they blood retest their hypothyroid patients, to see how thyroid hormone replacement is going. If retests are only done once-yearly or even twice, the TSH level (likely the one that was elevated when you were tested) can go up, indicating a need for a higher replacement dose to suppress the TSH level back down into the normal range.

As far as thyroid antibody levels go, these will fluctuate in autoimmune thyroiditis patients, throughout their lives.

The levels of them don't usually represent how well the hypothyroidism is treated. Some patients see them lower with hormone therapy but this is not always true. What I describe above has been the case with my treatment as a hypothyroid patient with Hashimoto's (thyroid antibodies are sometimes elevated, even with optimal treatment) and is how many medical sources also explain it.

Thyroid diseases run in families and some members may see hyperthyroidism develop from Graves' disease and from the antibodies that contribute to it (thyroid stimulating immunoglobulin "TSI"). Others have the antibodies that contribute to Hashimoto's being the "anti-thyroidperoxidase" (TPO) and the "anti-thyroglobulin" (TG). You might consider asking your doctor to go over your blood test results with you, to help you better understand these issues.

Eighty-Seven Thyroid Disease Questions Answered!

QUESTION SEVENTY-SEVEN

Is Blood Testing - A Doctor's Greatest Diagnostic Tool?

When I saw the first doctor for my thyroid symptoms, she diagnosed me with emotional only problems - "Generalized Anxiety Disorder". What puzzled me however was the fact that my very dry skin and joint/muscle aches that I complained about would also be considered emotional-only symptoms. I saw a different doctor to have blood tests ordered and my thyroid disease (hypothyroidism caused by Hashimoto's thyroiditis) was found.

I feel that due to doctors having problems with less-than detailed patients, who sometimes fail to fully relate their symptoms and doctors who may be overbooked and unable to spend as much time as needed with patients on certain days, blood testing should be resorted-to often. It is so incredibly diagnostic and only requires a stroke-of-the-pen to get them ordered.

I agree with the opinion that has been stated by medical sources, that lifetime viruses, allergens and environmental toxins can all cause our immune systems to go haywire over time and lots of medical research studies back this theory up. I have written on the fact that when a virus cannot be fully eradicated by the immune system, it may then resort to attacking the tissues in the body that contain them.

For these reasons, blood testing should be ordered for symptomatic patients who may have problems going on in their bodies that may not otherwise be diagnosed.

QUESTION SEVENTY-EIGHT

What Importance is there in Thyroid Antibodies Blood Tests?

In my lay opinion, but one that is based on lots of research on medical information sites and correspondence with literally 1,000s of fellow thyroid patients since year-2003, if thyroid disease runs in a family, "thyroid antibodies" test should also be tested for when blood labs are being done. These are the "anti-throidperoxidase" (TPO) and the "anti-thyroglobulin" (TG) and if either or both are positive, autoimmune thyroid disease is present regardless of thyroid hormone levels.

I have friends with Hashimoto's thyroiditis whose thyroid hormones were within normal range but their TPO antibody levels tested in the 1,000s. In some cases their doctors started them on thyroid hormone replacement therapy, which in some cases can slow down thyroid autoimmunity. Some of them were started on hormone therapy because thaey had mild to moderate goiters (thyroid gland swelling).

In my case for example - when I was diagnosed with hypothyroidism, my TSH was only moderately elevated @ "8.3" (normal range 0.4 to 4.5) and my thyroid hormones were only at mid-range or slightly below. At the same time my TG antibodies were @ "537" (range <40) so were almost 500 points above normal. My TPO antibodies were @ "120" (range <35). I was experiencing hypothyroid symptoms despite normal-range thyroid hormones. Your thyroid ABs may be negative but testing them will help rule out thyroid disease or confirm its presence.

QUESTION SEVENTY-NINE

Is My Hashimoto's Thyroiditis caused by Mononucleosis?

I too have Hashimoto's and treated for the hypothyroidism that resulted from it. I had mononucleosis at about age 10 and it was a severe case, keeping me out of school for six weeks. At age 40, both the thyroid disease and CFS (Chronic Fatigue Syndrome) manifested and my belief is that these can be traced-back to my bout of mono from the EBV virus.

Eighty-Seven Thyroid Disease Questions Answered!

When I was tested for EBV antibodies a few years ago, at my request, due to my thyroid treatment not alleviating the CFS symptoms, my result was "218" - the normal range being <20 (20 and above being positive). While 80% or more of the population has the EBV in their system, CFS and other autoimmune disease patients, including those with MS, often have very high titers of EBV antibodies (like mine).

This means the virus can remain in a highly replicated state in susceptible individuals (post viral illness) and medical research associates high titers with development of certain types of diseases and syndromes like CFS. This fact is also recognized by the U.S. National Institutes of Health.

QUESTION EIGHTY

Is Hypothyroid Treatment Available for Heart Patients?

Thyroid disease medical resources state that people being treated for heart conditions are usually replaced on thyroid hormone to correct their low thyroid hormone levels by suppressing the TSH level back down into the higher normal values range. TSH elevates with hypothyroidism and if the highest normal value for it at a blood testing lab is about 4.5 for example, the thyroid dose might only be adjusted to suppress the TSH back down to no lower than 3.0 or 4.0, within normal values. It depends on how severe your doctor determines your heart condition to be and how well controlled it is on your current treatments. Increasing the metabolism in the body via thyroid hormone can place added stress on the heart and is why it may be less-optimized in a heart patient than it would be in a patient with no cardiac issues.

QUESTION EIGHTY-ONE

What are the Pros and Cons of RAI Thyroid Gland Ablation?

After corresponding with literally 1,000s of thyroid patients since, year-2003, much of this being when I moderated patient-forums, lots of stories were related to me by patients who underwent RAI ablation, who had adverse reactions to it. Some saw a worsening of their "thyroid eye disease" for example, after weeks post-procedure. Others had successful ablations with no complications. This is why patients referred for the treatment should be thoroughly informed about risks and given the option of surgical thyroidectomy as an alternative choice (removal by surgery).

Thyroidectomies also have risks, such as inadvertent damage or removal of the parathyroid glands (these regulate calcium levels in the body) but if a patient has difficult-to-treat hyperthyroidism, they must undergo one or the other (RAI ablation or surgical removal). If severe hyperthyroidism is not treated and allowed to continue, heart problems and severe bone loss can occur.

These risks are also why I personally believe patients should first have drug treatment attempted (i.e. anti-thyroid drugs and/or beta-blocker drugs) before thyroid-removal options are offered. If these are not successful, then a choice has to me made between these other two options for gland removal. Lots of endocrinologists and thyroid specializing MDs agree with this opinion.

It is difficult if not impossible to fully cover a procedure like RAI in a single article and by attempting to do so, articles become too lengthy, so that readers seeking general info will bypass them. What one seeking information on this subject should consider doing, is writing down the "specific areas of information" you are seeking in regard to RAI and discuss those with your doctor or post them on a doctor-moderated forum, that has questions answered by a board certified endocrinologist or thyroid-specializing MD of some type.

QUESTION EIGHTY-TWO

Can Hashimoto's Thyroiditis go into Remission?

It is extremely rare for Hashimoto's autoimmune thyroiditis to go into remission and is in most cases, a life-long disease. The treatment is for the hypothyroidism it causes, once the antibodies that cause the disease have done damage to the thyroid gland and it no longer produces enough hormone. Replacement thyroid hormone drugs are the treatment and it is monitored via follow-up blood tests 1 to 3 times yearly. Some patients do not see complete relief of symptoms and sometimes, there is no explanation as to why this happens but it may be the disease aspect rather than imbalanced hormones, that contribute to ongoing symptoms.

Getting a replacement hormone dose best-optimized by the treating doctor is all that can be done. If one is taking a T4-only replacement hormone, they might consider asking their doctor to place them on a trial of combination T4 and T3 which gives better symptom relief to some patients.

While this is not true in all cases, it might be worth a trial if a doctor is willing. If other causes of symptoms are suspected, blood tests should be ordered to rule these out or to confirm them as co morbid conditions. This can be things like anemia, vitamin deficiencies, blood glucose imbalances and sex or adrenal hormone imbalances. Thyroid disease places these conditions at slightly higher risk for developing than in the general public, according to some medical research studies.

QUESTION EIGHTY-THREE

Should there be A Lowered Upper-Limit TSH Normal Values Range?

The NACB (National Academy of Clinical Biochemistry) and other medical groups have suggested the 2.5 upper limit cut off for blood TSH levels because if I remember correctly, they have found that 95% of the healthy population has a TSH normal value that is below 2.5, which would mean that levels at 2.5 and above can indicate developing hypothyroidism.

One medical research group that has published a study in regard to this suggested revision in the normal range, is the Journal of Clinical Endocrinology & Metabolism, in their article titled: "Upper Limit of Normal Serum Thyroid-Stimulating Hormone: A Moving and Now an Aging Target?"

This is an even lower upper limit than that suggested by the AACE ("3.0) and would likely detect more borderline and early onset cases as these medical groups are pointing out. If not for the AACE starting the ball rolling, labs would all likely still have the 5.0 and 6.0 upper-limit TSH value ranges.

QUESTION EIGHTY-FOUR

Could my Trembling Hands Indicate a Thyroid Problem?

An overactive thyroid gland (hyperthyroidism) can cause tremor, especially in the hands. A simple blood test called "TSH" (Thyroid Stimulating Hormone) can help to determine if you've developed a hyperthyroid disorder.

The TSH, which comes from the pituitary gland, rather than from the thyroid gland, begins to drop to low-normal, and below-normal levels with the onset of hyperthyroidism.

If you have the test ordered by your doctor and it's low or borderline-low, you could then have the actual thyroid hormones tested (T3 and T4) to see how severe the hyperthyroidism is. With the thyroid hormones, they do the opposite of TSH and elevate when the thyroid is overactive.

If hyperthyroidism is confirmed, a test for "thyroid antibodies" might also be needed, which are the cells from the immune system that attach to the thyroid gland, causing it to over-produce hormones. These are called "thyroid stimulating immunoglobulin" (TSI). If these are positive, Graves' disease (autoimmune cause) would likely be the diagnosis.

If you have hyperthyroidism there are treatments to slow the thyroid gland down and to treat symptoms of sped-up metabolism and the associated anxiety, nervousness and trembling.

Eighty-Seven Thyroid Disease Questions Answered!

Other than these suggestions, I would consider whether you have been taking any new supplements or drugs that might have a stimulating effect on your system, since this can be a cause of hand tremors as well.

QUESTION EIGHTY-FIVE

What Thyroid Test Result Indicates Hypothyroidism when Elevated?

That would be the TSH level (Thyroid Stimulating Hormone) and it is a pituitary hormone rather than a thyroid one but is very accurate and sensitive in reflecting how well the thyroid gland is functioning. It will actually become abnormal in early-onset thyroid disease cases, even before the thyroid hormones (T4 and T3) fall outside of normal values.

TSH begins to rise when the thyroid gland begins under functioning (hypothyroidism). Many blood testing labs have a normal-values range that is approximately from "0.5 to 5.0", so that anything above 5.0 is indicative of a hypothyroid condition.

Eighty-Seven Thyroid Disease Questions Answered!

Some thyroid specializing MDs and endocrinologists believe that a TSH at 10.0 and above, reveals "overt" hypothyroidism (full blown), regardless of where the T4 and/or T3 levels are at. With a TSH of "65" as yours is, your T4 and T3 are likely below normal and you are in need of thyroid hormone replacement therapy to correct the hypothyroidism. The treatment is simple and consists of taking a pill containing the proper dose-level of thyroid hormone to correct your low levels of them.

QUESTION EIGHTY-SIX

Why Do Treated Hypothyroid Patients have Weight Loss Difficulties?

I'm a male hypothyroid patient, so can give you an answer from personal experience. Also, I've know Mary Shomon for years, from the about.com thyroid disease site (great source of information).

I have also in fact, written reviews for her books, that she has sent me copies of, including "The Thyroid Diet".

I recommend you get a copy of that book, which you can find on a number of sources and the best booksellers, by doing a search using the title.

I too have had difficulty with weight loss since the onset of thyroid disease (hypothyroidism, caused by Hashimoto's thyroiditis). I am not terribly overweight but enough-so, that it places me at higher risk for things like diabetes. I don't mind relating my weight - which is 240lb at 6ft tall. I carry mine well because it evenly gains in my body, rather than just around my middle but I don't like the negative effect it has on my energy levels, so I am working hard on losing some pounds.

With us thyroid patients it just simply takes more effort to lose weight and to keep it off, than it does for the healthy public. My suspicion is that even treated hypothyroidism, still adversely affects bodily metabolism, subtly but enough-so, as to make it difficult to keep extra pounds off. You can probably find Mary's dieting guidelines in-summation at her about.com or her thyroid-info.com site, in addition to her in-print book.

You will increase your odds in successful weight loss and in maintaining it, if you seriously implement those as part of your treatment regimen. We must do our part, in addition to what our doctor is doing for us (be proactive).

Best wishes with it, from a fellow-patient who is rooting for you!

QUESTION EIGHTY-SEVEN

What are some of the Main Causes of Hypothyroidism?

Hypothyroidism can be caused by a number of things but in the more industrialized countries, the cause is "thyroid autoimmunity", also called "autoimmune thyroiditis" and "Hashimoto's disease". It is a process in which the thyroid gland becomes under active after being relentlessly attacked by auto-antibodies sent from the immune system that mistakenly identify it as an intruder, as it would allergens, bacteria and viruses.

Once enough thyroid cells are damaged by these antibodies over time, hypothyroidism sets in. In the less industrialized countries, where iodine rich foods are lacking or they do not have access to iodized sale, "iodine deficiency hypothyroidism" can be the cause. Other causes are things like a failure in the brain glands that regulate thyroid function (master-gland endocrine failure) which is called "central hypothyroidism". Women can develop a temporary form of thyroiditis when pregnant, that leaves them hypothyroid afterward, called "postpartum hypothyroidism" which can in some cases be temporary and other times permanent, needing lifelong treatment.

Some people are born with insufficient thyroid glands (small or partially missing) and as they enter their teens or adult years, their thyroid hormone levels become inadequate. This is referred to as "congenital hypothyroidism" and in some cases is diagnosed at birth and treated, with no negative consequences as the child develops.

People, who experience severe throat injuries, such as in car accidents, can damage their thyroid glands to the extent that they become under active.

Eighty-Seven Thyroid Disease Questions Answered!

And lastly, a person can experience hypothyroidism following exposure to chemicals or drugs that adversely affect the thyroid gland, called "chemical hypothyroidism". Lots of Russian people experienced hypothyroidism following the Chernobyl nuclear power plant accident in 1986, in which nuclear fallout affected their thyroid glands in years following, causing them to become under active.

At the basic level, an under active thyroid simply means one that is not producing enough hormone to properly regulate bodily metabolism.

(END)